The Easy Guide to

OSCEs

for Clinical Specialties

A Step-by-Step Guide to Success

Second Edition

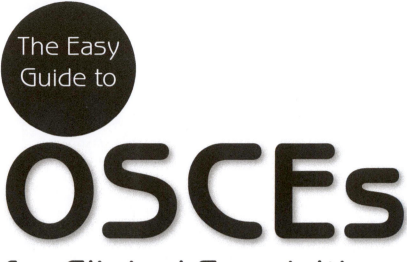

The Easy Guide to

OSCEs

for Clinical Specialties

A Step-by-Step Guide to Success

Second Edition

Nazmul Akunjee, MBBS MRCGP
GP Principal, North London

Muhammed Akunjee, MBBS MRCGP PgCert (Diabetes) PgCert (MedEd)
GP Principal, North London

Syed Jalali
Foundation Year Doctor, Cardiff

Shoaib Siddiqui
Foundation Year Doctor, Brighton

Dominic Pimenta, BSc (Hons) MBBS MRCP
Medical Registrar, London

Dilsan Yilmaz, BSc (Hons) MBBS MRCS
Academic Clinical Fellow in General Surgery, London

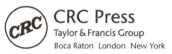
CRC Press
Taylor & Francis Group
Boca Raton London New York

CRC Press is an imprint of the
Taylor & Francis Group, an **informa** business

CRC Press
Taylor & Francis Group
6000 Broken Sound Parkway NW, Suite 300
Boca Raton, FL 33487-2742

© 2017 by Taylor & Francis Group, LLC
CRC Press is an imprint of Taylor & Francis Group, an Informa business

No claim to original U.S. Government works

Printed and bound in Great Britian by Ashford Colour Press Ltd, Gosport, Hampshire.
Version Date: 20160815

International Standard Book Number-13: 978-1-78523-120-9 (Paperback)

This book contains information obtained from authentic and highly regarded sources. While all reasonable efforts have been made to publish reliable data and information, neither the author[s] nor the publisher can accept any legal responsibility or liability for any errors or omissions that may be made. The publishers wish to make clear that any views or opinions expressed in this book by individual editors, authors or contributors are personal to them and do not necessarily reflect the views/opinions of the publishers. The information or guidance contained in this book is intended for use by medical, scientific or health-care professionals and is provided strictly as a supplement to the medical or other professional's own judgement, their knowledge of the patient's medical history, relevant manufacturer's instructions and the appropriate best practice guidelines. Because of the rapid advances in medical science, any information or advice on dosages, procedures or diagnoses should be independently verified. The reader is strongly urged to consult the relevant national drug formulary and the drug companies' and device or material manufacturers' printed instructions, and their websites, before administering or utilizing any of the drugs, devices or materials mentioned in this book. This book does not indicate whether a particular treatment is appropriate or suitable for a particular individual. Ultimately it is the sole responsibility of the medical professional to make his or her own professional judgements, so as to advise and treat patients appropriately. The authors and publishers have also attempted to trace the copyright holders of all material reproduced in this publication and apologize to copyright holders if permission to publish in this form has not been obtained. If any copyright material has not been acknowledged please write and let us know so we may rectify in any future reprint.

Library of Congress Cataloging-in-Publication Data

Library of Congress Cataloging-in-Publication Data
Names: Akunjee, Muhammed, author.
Title: The easy guide to OSCEs for specialties : a step-by-step guide to success / Muhammed Akunjee [and 5 others].
Description: Second edition. | Boca Raton : CRC Press, [2016]
Identifiers: LCCN 2016023637 | ISBN 9781785231209 (pbk. : alk. paper)
Subjects: | MESH: Clinical Medicine--methods | Problems and Exercises
Classification: LCC RC58 | NLM WB 18.2 | DDC 616.0076--dc23
LC record available at https://lccn.loc.gov/2016023637

Visit the Taylor & Francis Web site at
http://www.taylorandfrancis.com

and the CRC Press Web site at
http://www.crcpress.com

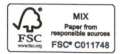

Contents

Contents

Preface to the First Edition

Following on from the unprecedented success of *The Easy Guide to OSCEs for Final Year Medical Students*, which was commended in the BMA Book Competition 2008, we have been inundated with requests from medical students and doctors alike to continue the series. This second book, *The Easy Guide to OSCEs for Specialties*, has drawn from and built upon the strengths of its predecessor and applied it to the diverse nature of medical specialties.

Specialties are playing an increasing role in the medical curriculum following the introduction of the foundation year programme. Junior doctors are now expected to be competent in a wide range of different skills in medical fields including obstetrics, paediatrics, geriatrics, anaesthetics and palliative care. For this reason medical schools are now standardising OSCEs in specialties and making them an essential component for qualifying as a competent junior doctor. Amongst medical students, OSCEs in specialty subjects are notorious for being the most difficult to prepare for due to the lack of a book dedicated to the subject. We have written *The Easy Guide to OSCEs for Specialties* to fill this void and ease the already burdensome workload of medical students.

The Easy Guide to OSCEs for Specialties has been compiled by recently qualified doctors who have experienced the new OSCE system first hand. Drawing on the success of the first book and taking into account feedback from students and doctors, this book has been written in a fresh style covering over 80 OSCE examination stations in a wide range of different subjects. We have maintained the style and approach of the first book, which was well embraced by medical students and examiners alike.

This book is unique in its own right, covering medical specialties including obstetrics, gynaecology, sexual health, paediatrics, dermatology, rheumatology, orthopaedics, emergency medicine, anaesthetics, geriatrics, patient discharge, palliative care, and the all-important communication skills. We have inserted a larger number of time-saving, student-friendly mnemonics, more vivid diagrams and extra clinical conditions to aid the revision process. We have also added end-of-OSCE station case summaries to simulate the information a student would be expected to glean and present to the examiners under exam conditions.

This book, in conjunction with its companion, *The Easy Guide to OSCEs for Final Year Medical Students*, should provide a step-by-step guide to OSCE success. We hope that these books will provide essential reading for medical students of all years and in particular help those who are facing the daunting prospect of OSCE examinations.

Muhammed Akunjee, Syed Jalali, and Shoaib Siddiqui
November 2008

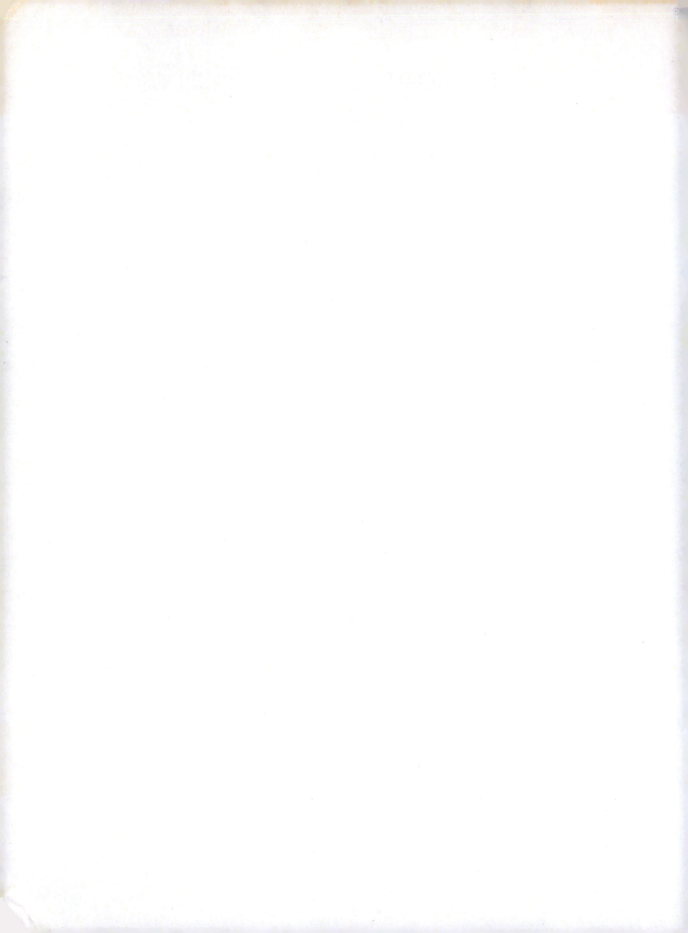

Foreword to the First Edition

End of year OSCE examinations for specialties prove to be a sticking point for a number of medical students, not least due to the vast array of specialty subjects students need to read, digest and practise, but also due to the lack of any single comprehensive text on the subject. *The Easy Guide to OSCEs for Specialties*, with its innovative approach, well-researched material and breadth of knowledge, provides the student with a firm foundation to tackle the often difficult OSCE scenarios head on.

In keeping with the approach of the popular *The Easy Guide to OSCEs for Final Year Medical Students*, this book maintains and improves on it in many ways. There are an increased number of vibrant illustrations, boxes of facts and differentials in addition to well thought-out, clinically-relevant case summaries.

The book also deals in depth with a wide range of difficult communication skill stations, giving students an excellent framework to approach such scenarios in full confidence, both under exam conditions and in real life.

We are sure that this book will be rewarding for medical students and examiners alike. We believe that it is essential reading for any student wishing to excel in their exams.

Graham Boswell MBBS FRCP
Consultant Physician
Medical OSCEs and PACES Examiner
Trust Foundation Programme Director, Hywel Dpa Trust

Steve Riley MB BCh MRCP MD Dip Med Ed
Consultant Nephrologist and General Physician University Hospital of Wales

November 2008

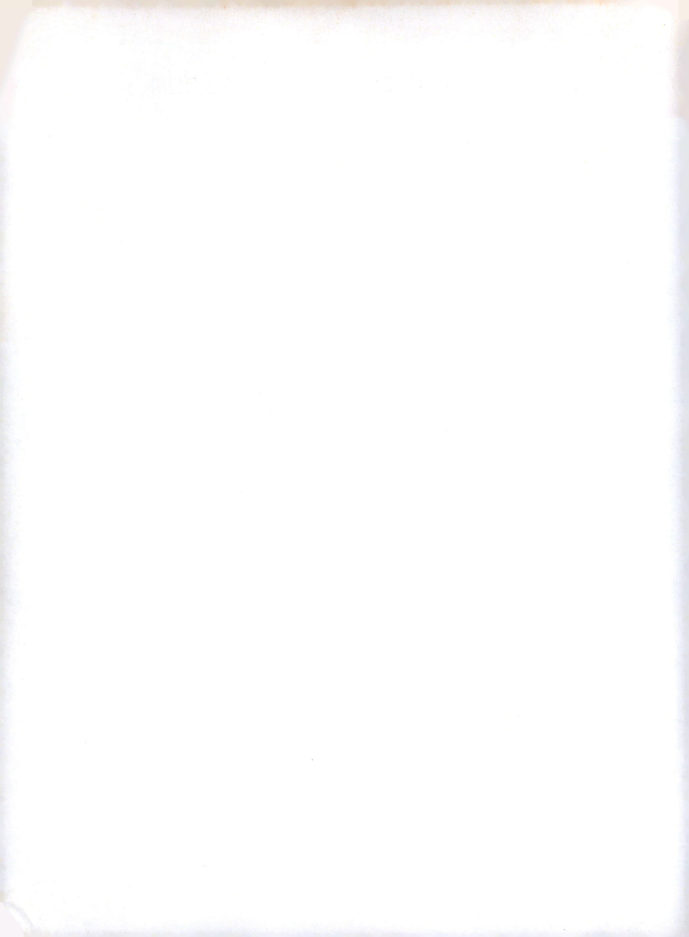

Preface to the Second Edition

Dear Reader,

Thank you for purchasing the expanded and fully revised edition of *The Easy Guide to OSCEs for Specialties*. We have worked hard to embody the principle of the editing authors, Nazmul and Muhammed Akunjee, to create a single resource with all the material a finals student could ever require to pass and excel in their OSCE exam.

The OSCE is the time to test your ability to behave and act like a doctor. You will find it is a culmination of all your knowledge, written and practical; and there is a third component: your evolving professional personality, that will be the seed that your career as a doctor will grow from.

For those of you just beginning your clinical training, this book will be an entry point to examining and to gaining practical experience. For those of you approaching finals, you already have all the knowledge you will ever need in your head. The secret to the exam, OSCE and written, is structure. By the end of the revision period you should be able to examine any part of the body, from top to toe, in a sensible manner without thinking about it.

This book emphasises the structure that you need to learn, as much as the individual steps, so that, as will be inevitable, when you find yourself presented with a situation you think you haven't prepared for, you will find that you actually have.

For those of you in between, keep going, and enjoy yourself! Medical school will be over far sooner than you think, or would like. Lastly, when you get in to the OSCE, remember finals is the time to transition into the doctor you want to be. So, stand up straight, stethoscope behind your back, and begin.

Good luck in your exams,

Dr Dominic Pimenta
BSc (Hons) MBBS MRCP, Medical Registrar, London

Miss Dilsan Yilmaz
MBBS MRCS, Academic Clinical Fellow in General Surgery, London

Mark Schemes

For each OSCE station we have defined a set of criteria which can be used when assessing oneself under examination conditions. The figures of 0, 1 and 2 indicate how many marks have been allocated for performing the task defined. Some criteria have been allocated two marks and this indicates that more than one task must be accomplished in those criteria to attain full marks. If only one task is completed, then a score of 1 will be attained. A score of 0 is given if the task was omitted completely.

Some OSCE criteria have no marks allocated. This is to reflect the fact that this is not a core competency skill, but that the inclusion of the task illustrates flair and higher achievement.

At the end of each OSCE station are five-point scales. The first indicates the examiner's mark for overall ability and the second five-point scale (in stations where role players are used) is for the role-player's overall assessment. A grade of 0 indicates an extremely poor performance, in which the candidate has not fulfilled any of the OSCE criteria, and has displayed poor communication skills and a lack of consideration for the role player's feelings. A grade of 3 indicates a fair performance, fulfilling most of the OSCE criteria and a grade of 5 is given to an exceptional candidate, who has fulfilled the OSCE criteria and performed the tasks competently and with confidence.

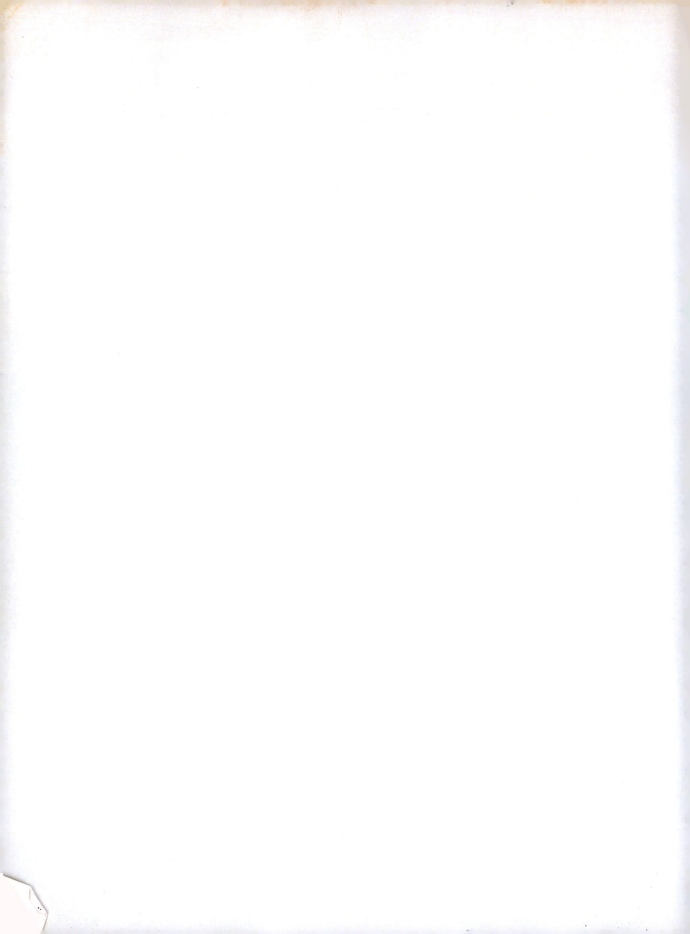

Obstetrics and Gynaecology

1.1   OBSTETRICS: OBSTETRICS HISTORY

INSTRUCTIONS

You are a foundation year House Officer in an antenatal clinic. Miss Newham has been referred to the GP for antenatal booking. Elicit a full obstetric history. You will be marked on your communication skills and your ability to take the history from the patient.

INTRODUCTION

1 2 3

☐☐☐	**Introduction**	Introduce yourself appropriately and establish rapport.
☐☐☐	**Name and Age**	Elicit the patient's name and age.
☐☐☐	**Occupation**	Enquire about the patient's occupation.

HISTORY

☐☐☐ **Concerns**   Elicit all the patient's presenting complaints. Use open questions and explore the patient's health beliefs. For each concern or complaint, elicit the patient's ideas, concerns and expectations.

'Good morning Miss Newham. Congratulations on your pregnancy. I hope everything is going well. How are you feeling today? Do you have any concerns about your pregnancy?'

☐☐☐ **History**   For each complaint, ascertain the time of onset, presenting features and associated symptoms. Explore each symptom systematically using appropriate mnemonics, e.g. SOCRATES (pain), ONE RESP (shortness of breath).

Questions to Ask in Vaginal Bleeding

Onset	When did it first begin? How long did you bleed for?
Frequency	How often does it occur? Has it happened in the past? Has it stopped now?
Volume	Did you notice any spotting on your clothes? Did you have to use any tampons, pads or sanitary towels? Were your clothes soaked? Were there any clots?
Pain	Is it associated with any pain (constant, colicky)?
Cause	Common causes of vaginal bleeding:
Early (< 24 wks)	Miscarriage, ectopic pregnancy, hydatidiform mole
Late (> 24 wks)	(*Antepartum haemorrhage*) Placental abruption, placenta praevia, uterine rupture

CURRENT PREGNANCY HISTORY

☐☐☐ **Present Preg.**   Enquire about the date of her last menstrual period (LMP). Establish the patient's certainty of the date, the regularity of her cycle and the typical cycle length prior to her LMP. Enquire about previous contraceptive use.

	Symptoms	Note for symptoms of pregnancy, including morning sickness, indigestion, urinary frequency and breast tenderness.
☐☐☐	**Gestation**	Calculate the number of weeks that the patient is pregnant and the estimated date of delivery. Ask the examiner for an obstetric wheel or use the formula below.

Calculating Estimated Date of Delivery

EDD = LMP – 3 months + 1 year and 7 days + (cycle length – 28)

	Complications	Ask if there have been any problems with this pregnancy, such as bleeding, spotting, or pain, or whether she is concerned about her blood pressure, her sugar levels or the baby's development. Has she had any recent urine infections or is she known to be anaemic?
☐☐☐	**Tests**	Enquire about the tests the patient may have had performed, including ultrasound scans (dating scan, anomaly scan or further scans for complications), Down's syndrome screening (blood test and nuchal scan), chorionic villus sampling and amniocentesis.

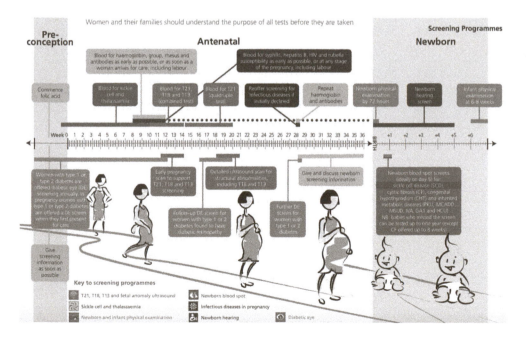

Fig. 1.1 © Crown Copyright 2013. This information was originally developed by Public Health England Screening (https://www.gov.uk/topic/population-screening-programmes) and is used under the Open Government Licence v3.0.

PAST OBSTETRIC HISTORY

☐ ☐ ☐   **Previous Preg.**   Ask the patient if this is her first pregnancy or if she has been pregnant before. If she was pregnant before, ask how many times she has been pregnant and whether she has had any miscarriages, stillbirths or terminations. Enquire about the gestations of previous pregnancies and the mode of delivery, i.e. was it spontaneous or induced, per vaginal (ventouse/forceps) or Caesarean section. If by Caesarean, ascertain the reason for this and whether it was an emergency or an elective procedure. Establish the birth weights of each child and whether there were any complications during the pregnancy or during delivery.

Common Obstetric Definitions

Gravidity	The number of pregnancies in total including any miscarriages or pregnancies lost before 24 weeks including current pregnancy
Parity	This is the number of potentially viable pregnancies beyond 24 weeks delivered not including the current pregnancy including stillbirths and livebirths
Para 3	Three term deliveries
Para 2+1	Two term pregnancies and a miscarriage at 20 weeks
Multiparous	Delivered live or potentially viable babies > 24 weeks' gestation
Nulliparous	Never delivered a live or potentially viable baby > 24 weeks' gestation

    Rhesus   Enquire about the patient's Rhesus status and whether she has received any Rhesus antibody injections.

ASSOCIATED HISTORY

    Gynae. History   Ask about the date and results of her last smear test (if indicated).

☐ ☐ ☐   **Medical History**   Has she had any operations or been admitted to hospital in the past? Does she suffer from any medical problems, including hypertension, diabetes, epilepsy, DVT or jaundice? Enquire specifically about thalassaemia or sickle-cell anaemia.

☐ ☐ ☐   **Drug History**   Is she taking any regular medication, prescribed or over-the-counter? Is she taking folic acid supplements and when did she start? (These should be started 3 months prior to conception and continued for 3 months into pregnancy.) Does she have any allergies?

    Family History   Is there any history of diabetes, high blood pressure or pregnancy-induced hypertension? Are there any congenital illnesses that run in the family? Is there any history of twin births in the family?

☐ ☐ ☐   **Social History**   Does she smoke or drink alcohol? Has she ever taken any recreational drugs? What type of accommodation does she live in and is anyone at home with her? Is she in a stable relationship? Will there be any help at home with the baby after delivery?

CLOSING

☐☐☐ **Rapport**   Establish and maintain rapport and demonstrate listening skills.
☐☐☐ **Summarise**   Check with patient and deliver an appropriate summary.

'This is Miss Newham, a 23-year old nulliparous woman who is currently 16 weeks pregnant. She is gravidum 2, parity 0 + 1 due to a previous termination of pregnancy at 12 weeks. She is currently happy with her pregnancy with no concerns and has been taking folic acid supplements up until 3 months' gestation. She suffers from no relevant medical illnesses or any allergies and is in a stable relationship with her boyfriend. She has no concerns but would like to know how many times she should visit the doctor and midwife.'

EXAMINER'S EVALUATION

1 2 3 4 5
☐☐☐☐☐   Overall assessment of taking an obstetric history
☐☐☐☐☐   Role player's score
             Total mark out of 26

DIFFERENTIAL DIAGNOSIS

Abdominal Pain in Pregnancy

The causes of abdominal pain in pregnancy can be classified according to the trimester in which it occurs. Non-pregnancy related causes such as appendicitis must also be kept in mind.

Causes of Abdominal Pain during Pregnancy

First trimester	Ectopic pregnancy (amenorrhoea, colicky and shoulder tip pain)
	Miscarriage (passage of products of conception, uterus normal size)
Second trimester	Miscarriage
Third trimester	Labour (contractions between 5–10 min, water breaks)
	False labour (irregular non-persistent contractions); pre-term labour (labour < 37 weeks)
	Placental abruption (dark painful blood, woody hard uterus)
	Uterine rupture (scarred uterus)
Other causes	Appendicitis, cholecystitis, GORD, urinary tract infection (UTI), gastroenteritis
Mnemonic:	'LARACROFT'
	Labour, Abruption of placenta, Rupture (ectopic, uterus), Abortion, Cholestasis, Rectus sheath haematoma, Ovarian tumour, Fibroids, Torsion of uterus

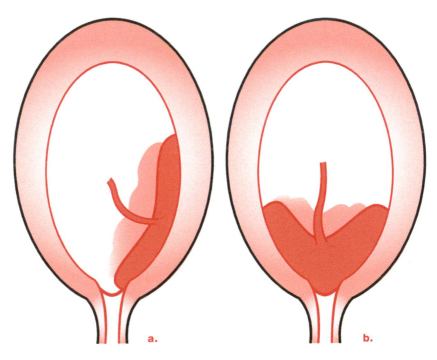

Fig. 1.2a and b Low-lying placenta with partial (left) and complete (right) obstruction of the internal os.

Placenta Praevia

This is when the placenta implants in the lower segment of the uterus, occurring in approximately one out of 200 pregnancies. It is usually more common in women who are multiparous, of increasing age and with uterine scarring following previous Caesarean sections.

Most cases are discovered on routine ultrasound examination as a 'low lying placenta', but a significant minority present with severe PV haemorrhage. Placenta praevia is classified according to the relationship of the placenta with the internal os. A marginal praevia is when the placenta is near or adjacent to the cervical os. However, if the placenta partially (Fig. 1.2a) or completely obscures (Fig. 1.2b) the internal os, this is known as major praevia. Such patients present with painless, bright red antepartum haemorrhage that increases in frequency and intensity over a number of weeks. The foetus may present with a transverse lie and breech presentation. A digital vaginal examination must *not* be performed in case massive bleeding is initiated.

Placental Abruption

This complicates 1% of pregnancies and occurs when part of or the entire placenta separates from the uterine wall before delivery, causing significant bleeding. Blood can track its way down the myometrium and presents as a dark, painful antepartum haemorrhage. However, in 20% of cases, visible vaginal blood is absent, known as concealed abruption (Fig. 1.3). On examination, the uterus is found to be tender and contracted, and in severe cases it may be woody and hard. The foetus may be difficult to palpate and foetal monitoring may show signs of compromise. There are a number of risk factors that predispose to abruption, including:

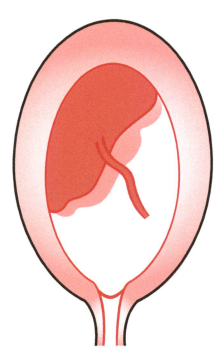

Fig. 1.3 Concealed abruption. Bleeding beneath the placenta causes disruption of the blood flow between the placenta and uterine wall, causing acute foetal hypoxia.

Risk Factors for Placental Abruption

MNEMONIC: PIPES

Pre-eclampsia
Intra-uterine growth restriction
Previous history of abruption
Essential hypertension
Smoking

Uterine Rupture

Uterine rupture occurs in approximately 1 in 1000 pregnancies. Although a relatively rare complication, it is often catastrophic in terms of maternal and fetal morbidity and mortality. It is important to note that there is a difference between rupture and scar dehiscence. The latter is more common and has a relatively better prognosis. Risk factors include previous uterine scar (previous Caesarean section or myomectomy), uterine trauma (blunt or penetrating abdominal trauma), overdistension of the uterus (polyhydramnios, macrosomia, more than one foetus) and obstructed labour.

1.2   OBSTETRICS: OBSTETRIC EXAMINATION

INSTRUCTIONS

You are meeting Mrs Foster for the first time. She is G4 P1 and is now 37 weeks pregnant. She has had her booking bloods and 20-week ultrasound scan, all of which have been normal. Please carry out an obstetric examination upon the patient and present your findings to the examiner as you go along.

NOTE

In the OSCE setting you may be provided with a dummy instead of a real patient. Ensure that you treat it with the same courtesy and respect as you would a real patient.

EXAMINATION

1 2 3

☐☐☐ **Introduction**   Introduce yourself. Elicit her name, age and occupation. Establish rapport.

History   Ask her whether she feels any foetal movements. Enquire about when they first started, their frequency and how many times a day she feels them, and whether they have changed in quality and quantity.

Consent   Explain the examination to the patient and seek her consent.

☐☐☐ **Chaperone**   Inform the patient that you may obtain a chaperone.

Position   Ask the patient to lie flat on the couch. Ensure that she is comfortable and expose her abdomen from the xiphisternum to the symphysis.

INSPECTION

☐☐☐ **General**   Stand and observe the patient from the edge of the bed. Look for signs consistent with pregnancy, scars, skin changes and foetal movements.

Signs to Observe in the Obstetric Examination

Symmetry	Symmetrical/asymmetrical abdominal distension
Scars	Pfannenstiel scar (low transverse scar from a previous C-section)
	Laparoscopic scar
Skin changes	Linea nigra (dark pigmented line from xiphisternum to the suprapubic region), striae gravidarum (purplish stretch marks denoting current parity), striae albicans (silver whitish striae denoting previous parity)
Umbilicus	Flattening, eversion (polyhydramnios, multiple pregnancy)
Movements	Foetal movements (occurring after 24 weeks of pregnancy)

PALPATION

☐☐☐ **General**   Enquire about pain before beginning the examination. Gently but firmly palpate the mother's abdomen. Note the uterine size, symphysio-fundal height, liquor volume, foetal movements, lie, presentation and uterine contractions.

☐☐☐ **Uterine Size**   Attempt to palpate the uterus and gauge its size. The uterus is palpable between weeks 12 and 14 and is level with the umbilicus by week 20. By week 36 the uterus is at the level of the xiphisternum.

        Amniotic Fluid   Estimate the liquor volume, noting for excessive amounts of fluid (polyhydramnios – gestational diabetes, foetal abnormality, idiopathic), reduced volume (oligohydramnios) or normal volume. Easily palpable foetal parts suggest reduced volume, while difficulty in palpation indicates increased volume.

☐☐☐ **SFH**   Establish the fundus of the uterus before measuring the symphysio-fundal height (SFH). Use the ulnar border of your left hand to find the fundus by repeatedly pressing on the abdomen from the xiphisternum downwards, until firmness is felt. Once the upper limit is established, place a tape measure, blind side up, measuring the distance from the fundus to the pubic symphysis. Turn the tape measure around to reveal the SFH in centimetres.

SFH Proportional to Gestational Age

The SFH provides an approximation of the gestational age in weeks. It is measured in centimetres from the symphysis pubis to the fundus. The margin of error increases with weeks of gestation

Weeks of gestation	Margin of error
20–36 weeks	+/– 2 cm
36–40 weeks	+/– 3 cm
> 40 weeks	+/– 4 cm

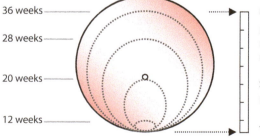

36 weeks
28 weeks
20 weeks
12 weeks

Uterine size
Fundus is palpable from 12–14th week
Uterus at level of umbilicus at 20th week
Uterus at level of the xiphisternum at 36th week

SFH (Symphysio-fundal height)
From week 20 the fundal height increases by 1cm / week and the SFH in cm approximates to the number of gestational weeks (up to week 36)

	Foetuses	Determine the number of foetuses present. Palpation of two foetal heads, a large uterus compared with gestation and auscultation of two separate foetal heartbeats with a variance of 10 bpm suggests the presence of multiple pregnancies.
☐☐☐	**Lie**	Palpate the foetal lie by facing the mother and placing one hand on either side of the uterus. Gently palpate down towards the pelvis. Determine the position of the foetus's back and limbs in order to ascertain its lie. Describe the lie as longitudinal, oblique or transverse in relation to the longitudinal axis of the uterus.
☐☐☐	**Presentation**	Turn and face the mother's feet. Firmly press above the symphysis pubis to determine the presentation. The presentation is the part of the foetus that presents first in relation to the pelvic inlet. Note if it is a cephalic (harder, rounder object on palpation) or breech (broader, softer object) presentation.
☐☐☐	**Engagement**	Engagement represents the amount of foetal head that has entered into the pelvis and is described in fifths of head palpable. It normally occurs after 37 weeks of gestation. It is an approximation of how many finger breadths of the head is palpable above the pelvic inlet. A foetal head that is more than 50% entered into the pelvic brim has only 2/5 of its surface area palpable abdominally and is engaged. If the foetal head is palpable by three or more finger breadths (i.e. less than 50% of the head has entered the pelvic inlet), it is not engaged.

Foetal head is not engaged and 5/5 palpable

Foetal head is engaged and 2/5 palpable

5 / 5 palpable
4 / 5 palpable
3 / 5 palpable
2 / 5 palpable
1 / 5 palpable
0 / 5 palpable

Degree of engagement of the foetal head

AUSCULTATION

☐☐☐	**Heartbeat**	Locate the anterior shoulder of the foetus and use a Pinard's stethoscope or sonicaid to listen for a heartbeat. If using the sonicaid, use ultrasound gel and wipe it off afterwards. Note the foetal heartbeat (normal between 110 and 160).

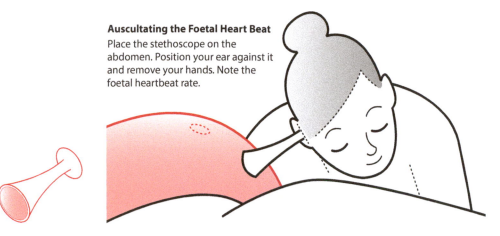

Auscultating the Foetal Heart Beat
Place the stethoscope on the abdomen. Position your ear against it and remove your hands. Note the foetal heartbeat rate.

Fig. 1.4 The wider hollow end is placed on the abdomen.

CLOSING

☐☐☐	**Oedema**	Check for the presence of ankle or sacral oedema.
☐☐☐	**BP**	Offer to check the mother's blood pressure (pre-eclampsia).
☐☐☐	**Urine**	Offer to check urine for proteinuria (pre-eclampsia) and glucose (gestational diabetes).
	Cover	Replace the woman's clothing.
☐☐☐	**Summarise**	Thank the mother. Answer any questions and summarise your findings.

'This is Mrs Foster who is currently 37 weeks pregnant. Her abdomen is consistent with a single uterine pregnancy and her SFH is 36 cm. The foetus is in longitudinal lie and is cephalic in presentation. The head is 5/5 palpable and not engaged. On sonicaid auscultation, the foetal heartbeat is 140 per minute with normal variation.'

EXAMINER'S EVALUATION

1 2 3 4 5
☐☐☐☐☐   Overall assessment of obstetric examination
        Total mark out of 22

DIFFERENTIAL DIAGNOSIS

Abnormal Lie

The foetal lie describes the position of the baby in relation to the longitudinal axis of the uterus. The foetus can be described as having a longitudinal, transverse or oblique lie. If the foetus is in a longitudinal lie, it can either be a breech or cephalic (head palpable in the pelvic inlet) presentation. In the oblique position the foetus's head or buttock can be palpable in either iliac fossa. In the transverse lie, the baby lies across the uterus with the head palpable in the flank

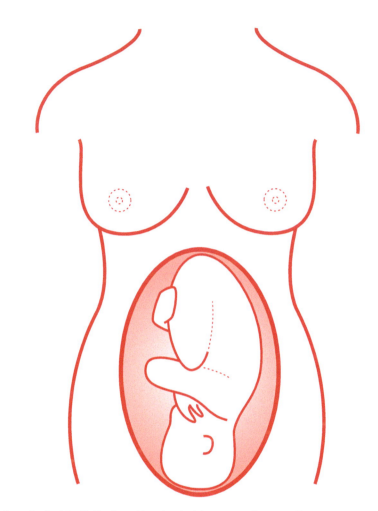

Fig. 1.5a Longitudinal lie. Buttock and head palpable at opposite ends. Presentation may be breech or cephalic depending on the presenting part.

and the pelvic inlet remaining empty. An abnormal lie is considered to be any position held by the foetus that is not parallel to the long axis of the uterus. Before 36 weeks an abnormal lie is common and is not predictive of the lie or presentation at the time of labour. On the other hand, an abnormal lie after 36 weeks is more likely to persist at the time of labour. It occurs in 0.5% of all pregnancies and is associated with pre-term labour, multiparity, multiple pregnancies (twins), polyhydramnios and placenta praevia. An abnormal lie is regarded as safe before 37 weeks, with the baby able to spontaneously progress to a longitudinal lie before labour. Beyond 37 weeks, an ultrasound should be carried out with a view to performing a Caesarean section.

Breech Presentation

The presentation is the part of the foetus that occupies the pelvic inlet. It can be either a cephalic or breech. A cephalic presentation is when the head is presented in the pelvic inlet, while a breech presentation is when the buttock is palpated instead, and the head is noted at

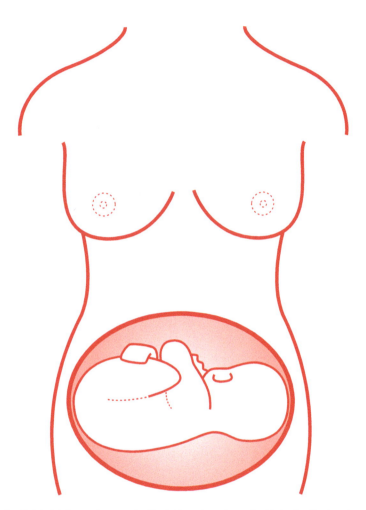

Fig. 1.5b Transverse lie. Pelvic inlet remains empty. Foetal hand maybe palpable in the flank, whereas in an oblique lie the head or buttock is felt in the iliac fossa.

the fundus. The incidence of breech presentations dramatically reduces through pregnancy, with up to 40% at week 20, falling to 3% at term. A breech presentation is only of concern after 37 weeks of gestation. An attempt at external cephalic version may be performed before considering a Caesarean section.

Breech Presentation

Associated conditions	Types of breech
Pre-term labour	Extended breech (baby's legs extended at the knees and flexed at the hip)
Multiple pregnancies	
Fibroids	Flexed breech (flexed at the knees and hips)
Placenta praevia	Footling breech (one or both feet found below the level of the buttocks)
Polyhydramnios	
Oligohydramnios	

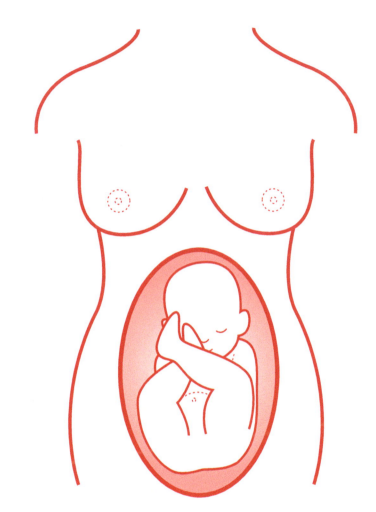

Fig. 1.6 Breech presentation: foetus is found in a longitudinal lie with the buttocks/feet facing down towards the cervix.

Multiple Pregnancies

Twins occur in 1 out of 105 pregnancies, with triplets occurring once in every 10 000 pregnancies. Predisposing factors include a family history of twins, an increase in maternal age, multiparity, in-vitro fertilisation and induced ovulation. Perinatal mortality increases with multiple pregnancies by a factor of four compared to singleton pregnancies. This can be explained by a higher incidence of miscarriage, pre-term delivery, intra-uterine growth retardation, congenital malformations and malpresentation. On examination, the uterus can be felt to be larger than expected for dates. There may be evidence of polyhydramnios, with more than two foetal poles and multiple foetal parts palpable. On auscultation, two distinct foetal heart rates can be heard, with a difference of 10 bpm between rates. The diagnosis can be confirmed on ultrasound. Features such as chorionicity and amnionicity (as demonstrated below) are established on ultrasound scanning.

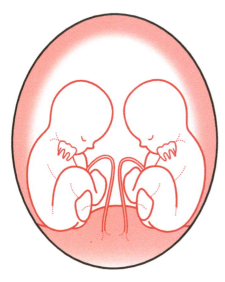

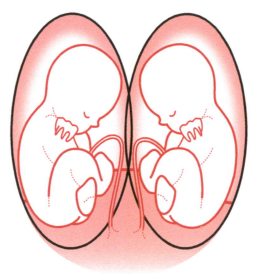

Fig. 1.7 Monochorionic monoamniotic twins – the twins share a placenta and an amniotic sac.

Fig. 1.8 Monochorionic diamniotic twins – the twins share a placenta but have separate amniotic sacs.

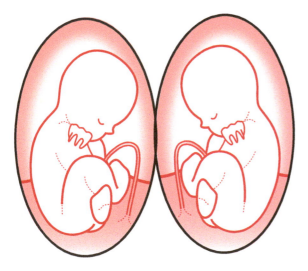

Fig. 1.9 Dichorionic diamniotic twins – the twins have separate placentas and amniotic sacs.

Abnormalities of the Amniotic Fluid

The amniotic fluid or liquor bathes the foetus in fluid, cushions it from trauma and promotes lung growth and development. The volume of fluid increases with gestational age, reaching a maximal volume of 1 litre by 34 to 38 weeks of gestation.

	Polyhydramnios	Oligohydramnios
Definition (both diagnoses are made on ultrasound)	Polyhydramnios occurs when the amniotic fluid exceeds 2–3 litres.	Oligohydramnios is suggested when the amniotic fluid volume is less than 500 mL at 34 weeks of gestation.
Clinical findings	The uterus is found to be oversized for the expected dates.	The uterus appears to be small for dates, with discrepancies in serial fundal height measurements. The foetal parts are also easily palpated through the mother's abdomen.
Causes/ associations	It can be due to impaired swallowing by the foetus or a blockage of the foetus's gastrointestinal tract. There is a strong association with congenital abnormalities such as oesophageal or duodenal atresia, Hirschsprung's disease, anencephaly, spina bifida and trisomy 21. Commoner causes include Type 2 maternal diabetes mellitus, multiple pregnancies and macrosomia.	It can be caused by the inability of the foetus to contribute to the amniotic fluid and produce urine (renal dysgenesis, polycystic kidneys, Potter's syndrome) or a rupture of the amniotic membranes.
Consequences	Polyhydramnios predisposes to pre-term labour, placental abruption and malpresentation.	It can result in the poor development of foetal lung tissue.

1.3   OBSTETRICS: URINE DIPSTICK AND BLOOD PRESSURE

INSTRUCTIONS

You are meeting Miss Paxter at an antenatal clinic. Please explain to the patient how to provide a urine specimen, and then dipstick her urine and check her blood pressure.

INTRODUCTION

1 2 3

☐☐☐   **Introduction**   Introduce yourself. Elicit the patient's name and age. Establish rapport.

DIPSTICK URINALYSIS

*Explanation

☐☐☐   **Fresh Sample**   Explain the importance of providing a fresh sample in the sterile container provided. Generally the urine sample should be no more than 4 hours old.

☐☐☐   **Cleaning**   Explain the need to clean the genitalia thoroughly with soap before providing a sample.

☐☐☐   **Mid-stream**   Explain to the patient how to deliver a mid-stream urine specimen and the importance of this.

'We need you to provide us with a fresh specimen of urine in this sterile container. So that we do not get any misleading results, it is important for you to clean and wash the area down below well, before taking the sample. Take the specimen bottle and sit as far back on the toilet seat as possible. Start to pass urine for a few seconds and when you are about halfway through, place the pot into the stream of urine and collect enough without overfilling it. Once you have done this please return the bottle to me.'

*Testing the Urine

☐☐☐   **Wear Gloves**   Wash hands and wear a pair of non-sterile gloves.

☐☐☐   **Test Strip**   Check the expiry date of the Multistix box and then remove a single testing strip, closing the lid immediately after doing so.

☐☐☐   **Dip**   Note the colour (cloudy/debris) and odour (pear drops – ketones, fishy – infection) of the urine. Place the whole stick in the urine for 1 second, ensuring that all testing areas are covered. Tap away any excess urine and hold the strip horizontally.

☐☐☐   **Results**   Read the stick correctly after 60 seconds or for the length of time indicated by the box.

☐☐☐   **Disposal**   Dispose of the soiled material and gloves in the yellow bag.

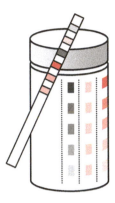

Dipstick Urine

Remove a testing stick, and dip into the urine sample for 1 second. Tap away excess and hold horizontally. Wait 60 seconds before interpretation.

*Closing

☐☐☐ **Explain**   Appropriately explain the findings to the patient.

Urine Dipstick Protein Analysis

Trace	Seldom significant
+	Proteinuria may be significant
++ or more	This is significant proteinuria and requires quantification within 24 hours of collection

☐☐☐ **Laboratory**   Mild proteinuria may be the result of a urinary tract infection. Even in the absence of nitrates or blood, request to send the specimen to the laboratory to confirm the presence of bacteria.

Check   Confirm that the patient has understood what you have told her.

'I dipsticked your urine and found some protein (+1). Often this may be simply the result of a urinary tract infection and hence I will be sending a sample to the laboratory to confirm this. However, on occasions, in pregnancy this may be due to raised blood pressure. Therefore I would now like to check your blood pressure to make sure it is stable.'

BLOOD PRESSURE

Note   It is important to select the appropriate cuff size to determine the patient's blood pressure. Cuffs that are too large for the patient's arm may result in a blood pressure that is lower than expected whilst cuffs that are too small may give a falsely elevated reading. The cuff bladder should have a width equal to at least 40% of the upper arm circumference.

☐☐☐ **Explain**   'Before I check your blood pressure, please could you sit up straight and remove your jumper. I will place a blood pressure cuff around your arm and inflate the cuff. This may feel a little uncomfortable. I will then place my stethoscope on your arm and take your pressure.'

☐☐☐ **Confirm**   Check that the patient has rested for at least 5 minutes.

*Procedure

☐ ☐ ☐	**Cuff**	Choose the appropriate cuff size for the patient.
	BP Machine	Check that the cuff is fully deflated and attached correctly.
☐ ☐ ☐	**Position**	Correctly position the patient with her arm horizontal and fully extended. Place the BP machine approximately in line with the level of the heart.
☐ ☐ ☐	**Placement**	Palpate the brachial artery and place the BP cuff neatly and securely around the arm above the antecubital fossa.
☐ ☐ ☐	**Check**	Check the approximate systolic level by palpating the radial or brachial artery once the cuff is inflated.
☐ ☐ ☐	**Procedure**	Auscultate over the brachial artery in the antecubital fossa and deflate the cuff slowly by 2–3 mmHg per second, watching the BP reading closely. Confirm the patient's systolic pressure by noting the pressure when the first audible Korotkoff sound can be heard. Note the diastolic pressure by the disappearance of the fifth Korotkoff sound (previously fourth in pregnancy – but there is no evidence to suggest this is accurate).

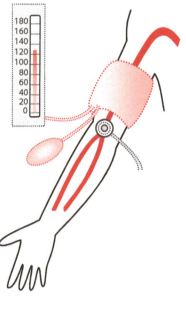

Measuring Blood Pressure

Choose the appropriate sized cuff. Feel for the brachial artery before placing the cuff around the arm. Listen with the stethoscope over the brachial artery while gradually deflating the cuff watching the BP closely.

☐ ☐ ☐	**Repeat**	Take at least two BP measurements.
☐ ☐ ☐	**Accuracy**	Ensure that the BP reading is measured to within 2 mmHg of the correct value.

*Closing

☐ ☐ ☐	**Interpreting**	Pre-eclampsia is diagnosed with a blood pressure reading of > 140/90 and a 24-hour urinary protein of > 0.3 g.

Indication for Hospital Admission

Symptoms	Signs
Headaches	Proteinuria of 1+ or > 0.3 g/24 hrs
Blurred vision	Diastolic blood pressure > 100 mmHg
Epigastric pain	Suspected foetal compromise

	Concerns	Deal with the patient's concerns appropriately and allay any fears.
☐ ☐ ☐	**Documents**	Ask for the patient's notes to document the BP reading.
	Questions	Thank the patient and ask if she has any questions.

EXAMINER'S EVALUATION

1 2 3 4 5
☐ ☐ ☐ ☐ ☐   Overall assessment of dipstick and BP check
Total mark out of 30

DIFFERENTIAL DIAGNOSIS

Urine dipstick and blood pressure testing are of great importance in pregnancy as they can indicate important treatable conditions which could otherwise go undiagnosed.

Pre-eclampsia

Definition	Characterised by pregnancy-induced hypertension (> 140/90 mmHg), proteinuria (> 0.3 g/24 hr) with or without oedema of the face, hands and feet.
	The term 'eclampsia' is derived from the Greek word *eklampsis*, meaning a 'sudden development' or a 'bolt from the blue'.
	It refers to convulsions that occur during pregnancy as a complication of pre-eclampsia.
Frequency	It affects approximately 7% of all pregnancies
Risk factors	More common in nulliparous women, those with a previous family history of pre-eclampsia, extremes of age (< 20 or > 35 years old), obesity, diabetes or hypertension.
Clinical features	It usually develops after week 20 of pregnancy and is resolved only by delivery.
	Other symptoms may include headaches, nausea and vomiting, epigastric pain and visual disturbances.
	Complications include eclampsia (grand mal seizures) that occurs in 1% of pre-eclampsia cases. Severe pre-eclampsia is defined as proteinuria, diastolic blood pressure > 100 mmHg or maternal complications.

Features of Pre-eclampsia

MNEMONIC: 'PRE ECLAMPSIA'

Proteinuria (> 0.3 g/24 hr)
Rising blood pressure (> 140/90 mmHg)
o**E**dema in the legs

Gestational Diabetes

Definition	Gestational diabetes is a temporary form of diabetes that affects pregnant women who have never suffered from diabetes before. It describes a transient elevation of glucose levels that disappears after pregnancy. It affects approximately 2% of all pregnant women compared to 0.3% of patients who have pre-existing diabetes.
Risk factors	A family history of type 2 diabetes, a previous history of gestational diabetes, increasing maternal age, obesity, ethnicity and smoking.
Clinical features	Include an increased risk of congenital abnormalities, pre-term labour, polyhydramnios and increased foetal mortality and morbidity. A glucose tolerance test will reveal an elevated sugar level (> 7.8 mmol of glucose) two hours after taking 75 g of glucose or a fasting glucose of > 5.6 mmol/L. Women who are diagnosed with gestational diabetes have a greater chance of developing diabetes mellitus later in life. **Foetal complications:** macrosomia, neonatal hypoglycaemia, congenital abnormalities (including cardiac defects), respiratory distress syndrome **Maternal complications:** increased risk of Caesarean section, pre-eclampsia, and type 2 diabetes

Urinary tract infection in pregnancy

Definition	Urinary tract infections affect 1 in 25 pregnancies.
Risk factors	Women are more susceptible to infections due to the close proximity of the shorter urethra to the anus. As a result, bowel organisms are able to ascend through the urethra (urethritis) and cause infection of the bladder (cystitis).
Clinical features	Symptoms include dysuria, frequency, urgency, nocturia, haematuria, suprapubic discomfort and tenderness, and cloudy or foul-smelling urine. A urine culture is often conclusive of a diagnosis but may take several days to process. Asymptomatic positive urine cultures should be treated with antibiotics in pregnancy. If nitrite or leucocyte esterase is positive, UTIs are highly likely. Often blood and urine protein are also detected. Up to 20% of untreated infections can lead to a pyelonephritis (fever, rigors, nausea, vomiting, loin pain). Premature labour is also a significant complication.

1.4   OBSTETRICS: NUCHAL SCANNING

INSTRUCTIONS

You are a foundation year House Officer in obstetrics. Mrs Lee is a 41-year old woman who is 8 weeks into her first pregnancy. She is due to have a nuchal scan, as part of her pregnancy dating scan, and would like you to explain more about this. You will be assessed on your communication skills and on the information that you provide.

INTRODUCTION

1 2 3

☐☐☐ **Introduction**   Introduce yourself. Elicit her name, age and occupation. Establish rapport.

☐☐☐ **Ideas**   Ask the patient what she understands by the term 'nuchal scanning' and what she thinks it will entail.

☐☐☐ **Concerns**   Ask the patient if she has any worries or concerns about the nuchal scan (e.g. risk of Down's, miscarriage). Make sure to explore these appropriately.

MEDICAL ADVICE

☐☐☐ **Screening Test**   Explain appropriately the purpose of the scan.

'The scan is part of an ultrasound screening test that is offered to all pregnant women to assess the risk of having a child with Down's syndrome, Edwards' or Patau's syndromes. It helps identify those mothers who may need more invasive diagnostic testing. The nuchal ultrasound test is safe and carries no risk of harm to yourself or your baby (such as miscarrying).'

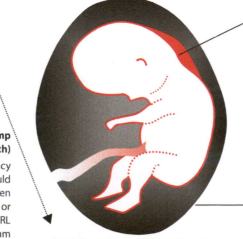

Nuchal Translucency

The area located posterior to the back of the skull and neck represents the nuchal translucency, which contains fluid. The widest part should be measured to evaluate the risk of developing Down's syndrome or a chromosomal abnormality. The diameter is normally less than 3mm. >3mm is considered abnormal and carries a 10% risk of an abnormality, while >6mm increases the risk to above 90%.

Amniotic fluid

CRL (Crown-Rump Length)

Nuchal translucency measurement should be obtained between 10 and 14 weeks or equivalent to a CRL between 45 and 84 mm

Nuchal translucency in Down's syndrome

☐☐☐   **Procedure**   Appropriately explain when the scan will be performed and what will be investigated.

'The scan will be performed between 10 and 14 weeks of your pregnancy. An ultrasound probe will be placed on your tummy along with some jelly. The dating scan will include measuring the thickness of the fat pad behind your baby's neck as well as other soft markers in the heart or head.'

☐☐☐   **Risk**   Explain how a risk ratio is arrived at.

'Along with the ultrasound findings, your general risk of having a baby with Down's syndrome or two other similar conditions is based upon your age and the results of the triple blood test. An overall risk will be calculated that represents the chance that your baby may have Down's syndrome or a similar condition. This figure will categorise you as being either at high risk (> 1 in 150) or at low risk (< 1 in 150). In some cases it is not possible to tell with the first tests alone and you will be offered further testing.'

Low Risk   Explain that being at low risk does not mean the baby does not have Down's, Edwards or Patau's syndromes.

'The nuchal scan as well as the combined blood test is the most effective non-invasive way of identifying Down's syndrome or similar conditions. However, it is important to appreciate that being categorised as "low risk" does not mean that your child definitely does not have Down's, but means that it is highly unlikely. You will be given a figure that represents the chance that your child will be affected. For example, a risk of 1 in 500 means that out of 500 births, one of these will be a Down's syndrome baby while the other 499 births will not.'

High Risk   Explain the procedure in the event of a positive result.

'If you are categorised as being at high risk (having greater than 1 in 150 chance that the child has Down's, Edwards or Patau's) then there are two options available to you. You can either choose to continue with the pregnancy without further investigation, or you may wish to pursue more invasive tests that check the baby's genes for Down's or similar conditions. It is important to remember that being told that you are at a higher risk does not mean that the baby definitely has Down's syndrome. This figure merely represents the probability that your child will be born with Down's. For example, a risk of 1 in 25 means that out of 25 births, one birth will be that of a baby with Down's syndrome.'

Association of Down's Syndrome with Maternal Age

Until recently, maternal age was the only factor used to identify mothers who are at high risk of developing a Down's syndrome baby. As demonstrated by the graph below, the risk of developing Down's syndrome increases exponentially with maternal age. Women aged over 35 are routinely offered invasive diagnostic tests. Recent studies have revealed that increasing paternal age also increases the risk of Down's, especially in older mothers.

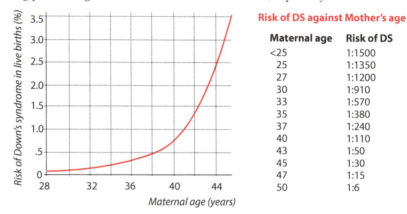

Risk of DS against Mother's age

Maternal age	Risk of DS
<25	1:1500
25	1:1350
27	1:1200
30	1:910
33	1:570
35	1:380
37	1:240
40	1:110
43	1:50
45	1:30
47	1:15
50	1:6

Assessing the Risk of Developing Down's Syndrome in a Baby

The overall risk value given to mothers takes into account a number of factors including the combined tests, maternal age, past medical and family history (genetic), crown-rump length and nuchal fold thickness (nuchal translucency).

☐☐☐ **Invasive Test**   Explain chorionic villus sampling and amniocentesis to the patient.

'We can take a sample from the placenta by passing a fine needle through the wall of your tummy. This is known as chorionic villus sampling and is carried out at 11 to 14 weeks of pregnancy. The other option, known as amniocentesis, is carried out at around 16 weeks and allows us to obtain the baby's cells from the surrounding fluid. Both of these tests carry a 1 in 100 chance of causing your pregnancy to miscarry.'

Pathology and Symptoms of Down's Syndrome

MNEMONIC: 'DOWN'

Decreased alpha-fetoprotein and unconjugated estriol (maternal)
One extra 21 chromosome
Women of advanced age
Non-disjunction during maternal meiosis

☐☐☐   **Follow-up**   Make appropriate arrangements to discuss results.

'The results are normally ready within 3–14 days of your test. The results are sent back to your doctor, who will make arrangements to discuss this with you. Please feel free to bring your partner or a family member with you for support.'

☐☐☐   **Pros and Cons**   Discuss the pros and cons of nuchal testing.

'Having the nuchal scan is very useful as it can reassure you as to whether your baby is likely to be healthy. It will give you the option to consider terminating the pregnancy if you so wish. If you decide to carry on with the pregnancy, it can give you time to prepare for the arrival of a baby with special needs. However, having a nuchal scan is not conclusive, as you may be categorised as being at high risk and yet go on to deliver a healthy baby. Hence, the procedure may cause undue anxiety and stress. If you have already decided that you want to keep a baby with Down's, Edwards or Patau's, then this procedure may result in unnecessary investigations. Here is some additional information about these conditions.'

         Summarise   Summarise back to the patient what you have explained so far.

CLOSING

☐☐☐   **Understanding**   Confirm that the patient has understood what you have explained to her.
☐☐☐   **Questions**   Respond appropriately to the patient's questions.
         Leaflet   Offer to give her more information in the form of a handout. Advise that the leaflet contains much of the information you have mentioned.

COMMUNICATION SKILLS

☐☐☐   **Rapport**   Attempt to establish rapport with the patient through the use of appropriate eye contact. Maintain appropriate body language and an open posture throughout.
☐☐☐   **Fluency**   Speak fluently and do not use jargon.
☐☐☐   **Listening**   Demonstrate interest and concern in what the patient says. Show active listening and listen empathetically.
☐☐☐   **Empathy**   Respond empathetically (offer emotional support and validate concerns).

EXAMINER'S EVALUATION

1 2 3 4 5
☐☐☐☐☐ Overall assessment of explaining nuchal translucency
☐☐☐☐☐ Role player's score
         Total mark out of 29

1.5 OBSTETRICS: BREAST-FEEDING

INSTRUCTIONS

You are a foundation year House Officer in general practice. Mrs Gillord is due to give birth to her first child in a few weeks' time. She has come to the practice as she is not sure whether to breast- or bottle-feed her child. Explore her concerns and give her appropriate advice. You will be assessed on your communication skills and on the information that you provide.

INTRODUCTION

1 2 3

☐ ☐ ☐ **Introduction** Introduce yourself. Elicit the patient's name, age and occupation. Establish rapport.

☐ ☐ ☐ **Ideas** Elicit the patient's ideas about breast-feeding.

☐ ☐ ☐ **Concerns** Establish any concerns or fears she has about breast-feeding her child.

Expectations Elicit how the patient would like to benefit from her consultation today.

ADVICE

☐ ☐ ☐ **Advantages** Explain the advantages of breast-feeding over bottle feeding for the child.

'We generally advise all our mothers to breast-feed their newborn children. This is because breast-feeding has a number of advantages over bottle feeding. Breast-feeding provides all the nutrients and energy that a baby needs in the first six months of life. It also includes antibodies to help protect the baby from infections and helps to maintain the growth and development of the baby. Recent evidence has shown that it helps prevent illnesses such as asthma, eczema and diabetes.'

Explain that breast-feeding has many advantages for the mother as well.

'Breast-feeding will have many benefits for you as a mother as well. It helps develop a strong bond between you and the baby. It helps the womb to return to its normal size quicker. This process uses up calories and so will allow you to return to your normal weight sooner. Breast milk is always ready and available when your child needs it and will not cost you anything. Also, recent evidence has shown that breast-feeding will help you in the long term. In particular, it helps to reduce your risk of developing breast and ovarian cancer.'

Benefits of Breast-feeding to Infant and Mother

MNEMONIC: 'ABCDEFGH'

Benefits to Infant	*Benefits to Mother*
Allergic conditions reduced	**E**conomical (free)
Best nutritional food for infant	**F**itness (body shape returns quicker)
Close relationship with mother	**G**uards against breast, ovary and uterus cancer
Development of IQ	**H**aemorrhage (postpartum) reduced

☐☐☐ **Disadvantages**   Explain the possibility of the transfer of infection and drugs to the baby while breast-feeding.

'Unfortunately along with nutrients, other substances can be transferred from mother to child in the breast milk. These include viruses such as HIV, and Hepatitis B may also be transmitted. Therefore if you are suffering from one of these illnesses you may be advised not to breast-feed. If you have had a breast reduction or breast implants, you will also not be able to breast-feed.'

'It is also important to realise that whatever you eat or drink may be passed to your baby through your breast milk. Such things include alcohol, caffeine and nicotine, which may harm your baby. Also, if you are on any medication or if you are going to start any new medication, let your doctor or pharmacist know that you are breast-feeding.'

Drugs Contraindicated in Breast-feeding

MNEMONIC: 'BREAST'

Bromocriptine, **B**enzodiazepines
Radioactive isotopes
Ergotamine, **E**thosuximide
Amiodarone, **A**mphetamines
Stimulant laxatives, **S**ex hormones
Tetracycline

☐☐☐ **Breast to Bottle**   Explain to the patient that breast-feeding should always be attempted before bottle feeding. This is because it is usually more difficult to switch from the bottle to the breast than it is from the breast to the bottle. Also remind the mother that it is often more difficult to restart breast milk once it is stopped.

☐☐☐ **Method**   Explain to the mother the technique required for breast-feeding. Encourage her to breast-feed soon after giving birth.

'During the latter part of pregnancy your breast will be primed to produce breast milk. Once your baby has been born this is a great time to start breast-feeding. This is because the first milk that you produce after giving birth will be extremely nutritious and beneficial to the baby.

'In order to breast-feed your child, you need to keep your baby's head and body in a straight line. Hold the baby close to you and keep the baby's nose opposite your nipple. Encourage the baby to latch on to your breast and hold the baby in a comfortable position. The more the baby sucks, the more milk is produced.

'I would like to reassure you that although this may sound tricky, most mothers find that breast-feeding comes naturally and as time goes by you will feel more confident. Remember that you can always approach your health visitor or your midwife for help and assistance.'

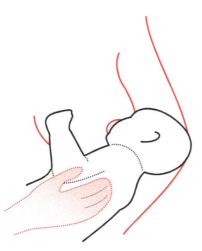

Breast-feeding Technique

Newborns commonly require on average eight feeds a day with each feed approximately 20 minutes in length. Hold the baby in such a way that her whole body is facing your body. Ensure that her nose and chin are pressed against your breast while supporting her head, neck and back. Allow the baby's mouth to latch onto your nipple and areola. If you wish to break the attachment, avoid pulling the baby away from your breast. Instead insert your little finger into the corner of her mouth and gently detach the baby from your breast.

☐ ☐ ☐ **Expressing**   Explain that breast milk can be given in expressed form.

Definition

'Breast milk does not have to be given only from the breast. You can also express it, which means squeezing the milk out of your breast with a pump.'

Reasons

'Expressing milk is useful for a number of reasons. Firstly, it can be used to give your child breast milk if it is it is having difficulty in suckling or when it is unwell and doesn't have enough energy.

'If your breasts feel uncomfortably full, you can express breast milk and store it to give to your baby later. If you wish to go back to work or are away from your baby, you can express milk so that your baby can still be fed breast milk.'

Method

'It is a good idea to ask your midwife or health visitor for advice.

'To express breast milk by hand, cup your breast and feel back from the end of your nipple to where the texture of the breast changes. From this area you need to use your thumb and index finger to gently squeeze toward your nipple. Milk should begin to flow at this point. This technique should become easier with time. Change to the other breast when milk stops flowing or slows down to a drip. If you are using a pump, please refer to the instruction manual.'

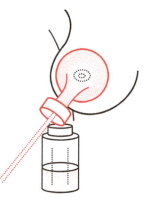

Using a Breast Pump

Breast pumps come in two varieties, hand and electric models. Ensure that the pump is sterilised before and after use. Breast milk can be frozen for a maximum of 3 months. Refer to the instruction manual regarding use of hand and electric models.

Storage

'Expressed milk can be stored in a fridge at a temperature of 2–4°C for 24 hours. It can also be stored in the ice compartment of a fridge for 1 week and for up to 3 months in a freezer. Always use a sterilised container for storage.'

☐☐☐ **Enough Milk**   Explain that there are certain signs that indicate the baby has had enough milk.

'You will know the baby has had enough milk as it will stop feeding by itself and appear satisfied after the feed. A well-fed baby should be gaining weight after 2 weeks and should wet around six nappies a day.'

	Other Fluids	Explain that other fluids should not be given during breast-feeding as this will reduce the amount of milk the mother will produce.
☐☐☐	**Dummies**	Explain that dummies should be avoided during the early months of breast-feeding as the baby may lose the ability to suckle the breast correctly.
☐☐☐	**Sore Nipples**	Explain that sore nipples can occur as a result of incorrect positioning during breast-feeding and that advice should be sought from the GP or health visitor.
☐☐☐	**Mastitis**	Explain and give advice regarding mastitis.

'Mastitis is when the breast becomes hot and tender and can be caused by infection. During this time you may also feel as though you have the flu. It is OK to carry on breast-feeding but you should get your midwife or health visitor to check your feeding position. If there is no improvement you should go to your GP as you may need a course of antibiotics.'

| **Duration** | Explain that there is no set limit to the time for breast-feeding. However, the mother should aim to breast-feed for between 6 and 12 months. The baby should be encouraged to eat solids after 4 months. |

Common Concerns during Breast-feeding

Breast size	Virtually all sizes and shapes of breasts can produce milk. After breast-feeding, some women notice that their breasts have become a little smaller or bigger. For other women there is no change.
From one breast	If there is only one functioning breast it is still possible to breast-feed effectively. If both breasts are being used, one breast should be drained completely before the other one is offered.
Refusal to feed	A baby's refusal to feed can sometimes be remedied by the mother simply resting and eating well before trying to feed the child again.
Sickness	If the mother becomes sick with a minor illness such as a cold or cough, it is usually fine for her to continue breast-feeding.
Alcohol	Mothers should be advised to avoid alcohol altogether while breast-feeding.
Pregnancy	Although breast-feeding significantly reduces the chances of pregnancy, mothers should be advised to used additional methods of contraception.

CLOSING

☐☐☐	**Understanding**	Confirm that the patient has understood what you have explained to her.
☐☐☐	**Questions**	Respond appropriately to her questions.
	Leaflet	Offer to give her more information in the form of a handout. Advise that the leaflet contains much of the information you have mentioned.

COMMUNICATION SKILLS

☐☐☐	**Rapport**	Attempt to establish rapport with the patient through the use of appropriate eye contact.
☐☐☐	**Fluency**	Speak fluently and do not use jargon.
☐☐☐	**Summarise**	Check with the patient and deliver an appropriate summary.

EXAMINER'S EVALUATION

1 2 3 4 5
☐☐☐☐☐ Overall assessment of breast-feeding advice
☐☐☐☐☐ Role player's score
       Total mark out of 31

1.6 OBSTETRICS: RASH-CONTACT COUNSELLING

INSTRUCTIONS

You are a foundation year House Officer in GP. Ms Franklin is 16 weeks pregnant and has presented having had recent contact with her neighbour's son, who has just developed chickenpox. Take a full history from the patient. Elicit her concerns and answer any questions she may have. You will be marked on your ability to elicit a relevant history and establish the risk to mother and foetus.

INTRODUCTION

1 2 3
☐☐☐ **Introduction** Introduce yourself. Elicit the patient's name and age, and age of pregnancy. Establish rapport.

HISTORY

☐☐☐ **Concerns** Elicit all the patient's presenting concerns. Use open questions and explore the patient's beliefs about their health. For each concern or complaint, elicit the patient's ideas, concerns and expectations.

☐☐☐ **History** Risk
Establish the patient's pre-existing risk:
- Ask about booking bloods (see below).
- Ask about personal history of chickenpox.
- Ask about immunisation history.
- Ask about other children at home, their age, and their chickenpox status.

☐☐☐ **Exposure** Establish the patient's exposure to the contact:
- Ask about age of exposure contact – in this case the neighbour's son.
- Ask about timing of exposure in relation to outbreak of the rash.
- Ask about the rash – maculopapular or vesicular.
- Ask about length of exposure and type – kissing contact, touching, shared room space only, etc.

ASSOCIATED HISTORY

☐☐☐ **Obstetric History** 'Do you have any children? How many? What type of delivery did they have? Have you had any miscarriages or terminations?'

☐☐☐ **Medical History** 'Do you suffer from any medical illness? Have you ever been admitted to hospital?' Ask specifically about immunisations and chickenpox history if you have not done so already.

☐☐☐ **Drug History** 'Do you take any medications?'

☐☐☐ **Social History** 'Do you smoke? Do you drink alcohol? Do you take recreational drugs?'

EXPLAIN

Explain correctly the risk of infectious period in chickenpox (from 48 hours prior to rash appearance until all papules have fully crusted over).

Explain correctly the risk to the foetus – a small risk of foetal varicella malformations in the first trimester. A risk of peripartum varicella zoster infection in the last trimester.

Explain correctly the risk to the mother – highest risk to the mother in the first trimester of pregnancy with varicella pneumonitis.

Explain correctly the treatment – for any significant risk in a non-immune individual in the first trimester, presenting early, varicella zoster immunoglobulin should be given. For any immune individual there is no need for treatment. The importance of monitoring for rash, shortness of breath and urgent care referral should be emphasised.

COMMUNICATION SKILLS

☐☐☐ **Rapport** Establish and maintain rapport with the patient and demonstrate listening skills.

☐☐☐ **Response** React positively to and acknowledge the patient's emotions.

☐☐☐ **Fluency** Speak fluently and do not use jargon.

☐☐☐ **Summarise** Check with the patient and deliver an appropriate summary.

'This is Ms Franklin, who is 16 weeks pregnant with her second pregnancy, and has a 2-year-old boy at home. She came into contact with her neighbour's son yesterday, spent 45 minutes in the same room while visiting the child, and may have had a limited kissing contact. She does not recall ever having chickenpox herself, nor has her child. She has had her antenatal screening bloods sent – all were negative. ToRCH screen bloods sent after contact, but she does not have the results. Her neighbour's son developed the chickenpox papules this morning. She is otherwise fit and well, works as a kindergarten teacher and feels completely well. I have advised her the risk to the foetus and mother is slim at 16 weeks, but we would need to speak with a obstetrics specialist early and get varicella immunoglobulin if authorised.'

EXAMINER'S EVALUATION

1 2 3 4 5

☐☐☐☐☐ Overall assessment of rash contact counselling

☐☐☐☐☐ Role player's score

Total mark

DIFFERENTIAL DIAGNOSIS

Overall Assessment

It is important to know several pregnancy-related risk infections and how to manage them, plus the possible risk to the foetus.

Antenatal Screening for Infectious Diseases

NICE recommends routine screening for infectious disease, now consisting of HIV, Hepatitis B, Rubella and syphilis before 10 weeks.

Herpes, toxoplasma and CMV are not recommended routinely, these are sent for if symptoms are identified during pregnancy or an abnormality is detected in utero – this is a ToRCH screen.

Congenital Varicella Syndrome

Includes skin scarring or loss, loss of limbs, neurological deficit, microcephaly and opthalmological defects. Greatest risk in the 1st trimester.

Congenital Rubella Syndrome

Diagnosis is a triad of deafness, ophthalmic and cardiac defects. Intellectual and physical disability are occasionally associated.

Congenital Syphilis

Very rare – symptoms can be divided into at-birth, early and late congenital syphilis. At-birth symptoms include skin lesions, deafness, prematurity, skeletal abnormalities. Untreated early syphilis can progress to late congenital syphilis – Hutchinson's teeth, deafness, saber shins and saddle nose and keratitis are the common features.

Infections During Pregnancy

Infection	Infectious period	Significant exposure	Risk to the foetus	Risk to the mother	Treatment
Varicella zoster (chickenpox, shingles)	48 hours prior to rash until papules completely crusted over. Incubation is 10–21 days.	Any kissing contact. > 30 minutes in the same room.	1st trimester: congenital varicella zoster (see below). 2nd–3rd trimester: shingles infancy. Peripartum-neonatal varicella.	1st trimester: varicella pneumonitis (which can be life-threatening)	Urgent varicella IgG screen. For non-immune: Varicella IVIG can be given with the first 72 hours of contact. Post-natal vaccination.
Rubella	7d before rash to 10d after. Incubation 10–21d.	Any kissing contact. > 30 minutes in the same room.	1st trimester: high risk of congenital rubella syndrome (see above). 2nd trimester: 20% congenital rubella syndrome, later, small risk of deafness. 3rd trimester: no risk.	Nil significant	Urgent rubella IgG screen (part of the booking bloods) For non-immune: No treatment Post-natal MMR vaccine
Parvovirus B19 'slapped cheek rash'	10d before rash to rash onset	Any kissing contact. > 30 minutes in the same room.	Small chance of excess foetal loss < 20 weeks	Nil	None
Measles	4d before to 4d after rash onset, incubation 7–18d	Any kissing contact. > 30 minutes in the same room (during infectious period).	Excess foetal loss. Perinatal: neonatal measles.	Severe pneumonitis	Check measles IgG. Give human normal IgG if within 6d of contact. Post-natal MMR.

1.7   OBSTETRICS: OBSTETRIC EMERGENCIES

POSTPARTUM HAEMORRHAGE

You are called for help by a midwife who is with a 35-year-old woman who has just delivered baby and placenta via normal vaginal delivery. She is gravida 4 para 4. You are told she has lost over 1000 mL of blood. Please assess and manage her.

Stage	Key points and actions	Score
Danger	Checks around the bedside for potential hazards; e.g. spills, wires, blood	
Response	Introduce yourself. Ask a simple question	
Airway	Recognise airway patency as patient is speaking	
Breathing		
	Look for signs of respiratory distress	
Measure	Respiratory rate	
	Saturations	
Treat	High flow oxygen	
Circulation		
Look	Assess the amount of blood, soaked sheets/swabs or clots present	
Feel	Volume of pulses	
Listen	Auscultation of heart sounds	
Measure	Heart rate	
	Blood pressure	
	Temperature	
Treat	Intravenous access and send bloods for FBC, U&Es, group and cross match, clotting	
	Warming measures (as available)	
	State that you would infuse blood as soon as possible and put out major haemorrhage call	
	State that whilst blood is being organised you would give IV fluid	
	Urethral catheterisation	
Disability	AVPU	
	Blood sugar measurement	
Exposure	Ensure patient is adequately exposed and that the source of bleeding can be identified	
Causes of postpartum haemorrhage to be considered	The 4 Ts: • Tone (abnormalities of uterine contraction) • Tissue (retained products of conception) • Trauma (of the genital tract) • Thrombin (abnormalities of coagulation)	

Postpartum haemorrhage is an important cause of maternal morbidity and mortality. It must be recognised and treated promptly. The Royal College of Obstetricians provide a very clear guideline on the management of PPH: www.rcog.org.uk/globalassets/documents/guidelines/gt52postpartumhaemorrhage0411.pdf.

As a junior doctor you should be able to provide the initial management as outlined for above and call for the appropriate help. Understanding the risk factors of PPH and being able to state the management of uterine atony (the most common cause of PPH) is important.

Risk factors for PPH

Antenatal risk factors		Risk factors identifiable during labour (Four Ts = tone, thrombin, tissue, trauma)
Maternal factors:	Pregnancy factors:	Tone: uterine atony, distended bladder
Age over 40	Placental abruption	Thrombin: pre-existing or acquired coagulopathy
Asian ethnicity	Placenta praevia	Tissue: retained placenta or clots
Obesity (BMI > 35)	Multiple pregnancy	Trauma: lacerations uterus, cervix or vagina
Anaemia (< 9 g/dl)	Pre-eclampsia	+induction of labour
	Gestational diabetes	

1.8   GYNAECOLOGY: GYNAECOLOGICAL HISTORY

INSTRUCTIONS

You are a foundation year House Officer in an outpatient gynaecology clinic. Mrs Paborski, a 59-year-old woman, presents to you for the first time complaining of heavy vaginal bleeding. Take a full gynaecological history from the patient.

INTRODUCTION

1 2 3

☐☐☐ **Introduction**   Introduce yourself appropriately and establish rapport.
☐☐☐ **Name and Age**   Elicit the patient's name and age.
☐☐☐ **Occupation**   Enquire about the patient's occupation.

HISTORY

☐☐☐ **Concerns**   Elicit all the patient's presenting concerns. Use open questions and explore the patient's beliefs about her health. For each concern or complaint, elicit the patient's ideas, concerns and expectations.

☐☐☐ **History**   For each complaint, ascertain the time of onset, presenting features and associated symptoms. Explore each symptom systematically using appropriate mnemonics, e.g. SOCRATES (pain), ONE RESP (shortness of breath).

GYNAECOLOGICAL HISTORY

☐☐☐ **Periods**   Establish the patient's age of menarche (first menstrual period). Enquire about the date of her last menstrual period (LMP), its duration and regularity. Ask if she has noticed any heavy bleeding (menorrhagia) and how much. Does she use tampons, pads or sanitary towels? Were they soaked and how many did she use? Did she soil her underwear? Were there any clots?

Causes of Vaginal Bleeding in a Non-Pregnant Woman

General	Thyroid disease, hepatic disorders, leukaemia and myeloproliferative disorders, thrombocytopenia, coagulopathies
Local	Vaginitis, fibroids, polyps, adenomyosis, endometriosis, infection (chlamydia, gonorrhoea), tumours (ovarian, endometrial and cervical), foreign body, trauma
Other	Dysfunctional uterine bleeding (DUB): no anatomical or systemic cause is found, foreign body (tissue paper), trauma (abuse)

☐☐☐ **Irregular Bleed**   Enquire about bleeding between periods (inter-menstrual) and following sexual intercourse (post-coital).

Causes of Inter-menstrual (IMB) and Post-coital bleeding (PCB)

IMB	Vaginal bleeding occurring in the menstrual cycle other than normal menstruation
Physiological	1–2% women spot around ovulation
Obstetric	Pregnancy, ectopic pregnancy, gestational trophoblastic disease
Uterine	Endometrial polyps, endometrial carcinoma, adenomyosis, fibroids
Vaginal	Vaginitis, vaginal malignancy
Cervical	Cervical cancer (commonly post-coital), cervical polyps, ectropion, cervicitis (blood-tinged discharge)
Iatrogenic	Contraceptive pills, tamoxifen, anticoagulants, SSRIs, corticosteroids
PCB	Vaginal bleeding that occurs immediately after sexual intercourse
Causes	Cervicitis, cervical and endometrial polyps, vaginal cancer, cervical cancer, infection (Chlamydia, gonorrhoea, trichomoniasis, yeast), trauma

☐☐☐ **Menopause**   Establish if the patient is menopausal. If so, ask for how long she has been menopausal and if she has had any post-menopausal bleeding.

Causes of Post-Menopausal Bleeding (PMB)

PMB	Vaginal bleeding 6 months after menopause. Any PMB should be treated as malignant until proved otherwise
Causes	Atrophic vaginitis (90%), infections (chlamydia, gonorrhoea, trichomoniasis), polyps (cervical or endometrial), endometrial carcinoma, cervical carcinoma, ovarian carcinoma, vaginal carcinoma, uterine sarcoma
Other	Hormone replacement therapy (HRT), clotting disorder, trauma

☐☐☐ **Pain**   Note any associated pain during her periods (dysmenorrhoea), particularly the timing in the cycle, its location, duration, radiation and severity. Note any other associated symptoms.

ASSOCIATED HISTORY

☐☐☐ **Sexual History**   Establish if the patient is sexually active. Is she suffering from any dyspareunia (if so, is the pain superficial or deep)? Is she with a regular sexual partner?

Discharge   Enquire if she is experiencing any vaginal discharge. Note its colour (clear, white, purulent, bloodstained), odour and amount. Is there associated pruritus? Is the partner experiencing any symptoms?

Gynae. History   Enquire about the date and result of her previous smear test. Did she have any previous abnormal results, if so, what was done (colposcopy)? Establish if the patient is using contraception (barrier methods, the pill, intramuscular contraception, the coil) and enquire about her current method.

OTHER ASSOCIATED HISTORY

☐☐☐ **Obstetric History** Has she ever been pregnant? If so, how many times and what were their gestations? Has she had any terminations of pregnancy, stillbirths or miscarriages?

Medical History Has she had any previous surgery or any serious illnesses (e.g. breast, cervical or ovarian cancer)?

☐☐☐ **Family History** Is there any history of any serious medical illness in the family such as breast or ovarian cancer? Enquire about the ages of the family member at the onset of such illnesses.

☐☐☐ **Drug History** Is she taking any regular medications (tamoxifen, OCP, HRT), prescribed or over the counter? Does she have any allergies?

Risk Factors for Endometrial Carcinoma

MNEMONIC: 'ENDOMET'

Elderly
Nulliparity
Diabetes
Obesity
Menstrual irregularity
o**E**strogen therapy
hyper**T**ension

Social History Does she drink alcohol or smoke?

Systemic Review Does she have any constitutional symptoms, such as weight loss, loss of appetite, increased fatigue, sweating and hot flushes? Does she suffer from any urinary symptoms, such as abdominal pain or dysuria?

Questions to Ask about Urinary Symptoms

Pain	Have you experienced any pain passing water (dysuria) or pain in your loins?
Frequency	How frequently do you pass water (frequency > 6/day)?
Nocturia	Do you ever go during the night (nocturia > 2/night)?
Urgency	Do you have a strong desire to pass urine (urgency)? Have you ever had accidents (bedwetting – enuresis)?
Straining	Do you have episodes of incontinence with straining or coughing (stress)? Do you ever leak when you are just walking? Do you use pads to keep yourself dry? How many do you use in a day?
Haematuria	Have you noticed any blood in your urine?
Other	Associated fever? Do you have any sensation of a mass in your vagina or a dragging heavy sensation (prolapse)?

CLOSING

□□□ **Rapport** Establish and maintain rapport and demonstrate listening skills.
□□□ **Summarise** Check with patient and deliver an appropriate summary.

'This is Mrs Paborski, a 59-year-old Polish woman with a three-months' history of vaginal bleeding. Her last LMP was 7 years ago. She states that the bleeding is progressively worsening, and has been occurring on a daily basis for the past 2 weeks. She has no abdominal pain but mentions that she has been unintentionally losing weight. She has been using HRT for the last 5 years but was stopped by her GP 2 months ago. In view of her gynaecological history, I suspect that this may be a case of endometrial cancer and I would like to perform a full pelvic examination, including a smear. I would also like to refer her for an urgent transvaginal ultrasound and hysteroscopy with biopsy, if indicated.'

EXAMINER'S EVALUATION

1 2 3 4 5
□ □ □ □ □ Overall assessment of gynaecological history-taking
□ □ □ □ □ Role player's score
Total mark out of 28

DIFFERENTIAL DIAGNOSIS

Menopause

In the UK the average age of menopause is between 51 and 52 years of age. It is usually preceded by the climacteric, which is a transitional phase in which there is an irregular response of the ovaries to pituitary stimuli, manifesting as erratic ovulation and menstruation. Menopause before 40 years of age is considered premature. In the early stages of the menopause, a woman may experience a number of symptoms such as hot flushes, insomnia, poor concentration, fatigue, vaginal dryness and a reduced libido.

Amenorrhoea

Amenorrhoea is defined as the absence of a menstrual period in a woman of reproductive age. It is derived from the Greek word *amenorroia*, which means 'a lack of monthly flow'. It becomes clinically significant when there is a failure of menstruation lasting longer than 6 months (or six cycles) in a woman of reproductive age (16–40 years) who is not pregnant. It is subdivided into primary and secondary amenorrhoea, depending on the time of onset. Primary amenorrhoea is the complete absence of menses in a 14-year-old with a lack of secondary sexual characteristics or in a 16-year-old with a normal development of sexual characteristics. Secondary amenorrhoea is the cessation of menstruation in a patient who has had periods previously for at least 6 months. Amenorrhoea can be normal in prepubertal girls, during pregnancy, lactation, postmenopause and as a result of contraception.

Causes of Amenorrhoea

Primary	Absence of menses by 14 years with lack of 2° sexual characteristics or by 16 years with normal 2° sexual characteristics
Familial	Constitutional delay (FH)
Structural	Imperforate hymen, haematocolpos
Genetic	Turner's syndrome, Prader–Willi syndrome
Congenital	Testicular feminisation
Organic	Hypo/hyperthyroidism, adrenal tumours/hyperplasia, PCOS
Other	Anorexia nervosa, psychological, athleticism, drugs (oral contraceptives)
Secondary	Cessation of menstruation with no periods for at least 6 months
Hypothalamic	Hypogonadism (Kallmann's syndrome), anorexia nervosa
Pituitary	Hyperprolactinaemia (pituitary hyperplasia/adenoma), Sheehan's syndrome
Ovary	Premature menopause, PCOS, ovarian dysgenesis (Turner's)
Other	Thyroid (hypo/hyperthyroidism), adrenal (hyperplasia, Cushing's syndrome, advanced Addison's disease), pancreas (diabetes)

Menorrhagia

Menorrhagia is defined as the loss of more than 80 mL of blood per cycle. It is often used to describe blood loss that has lasted longer than 7 days. Menstrual periods on average are expected to last a maximum of 5 days, with total blood flow of between 25 and 80 mL. Apart from heavy bleeding, patients may complain of symptoms of anaemia. Causes can be both local and systemic (thyroid disease and clotting disorders). However, in around 60% of cases no abnormality can be found and this is known as dysfunctional uterine bleeding. Patients often complain of having to make increased use of sanitary towels or tampons, and they may experience floods or pass clots. Bleeding associated with secondary dysmenorrhoea, which occurs several days before the onset of menstruation, may be indicative of fibroids, endometriosis, adenomyosis or ovarian tumours.

Causes of Menorrhagia

Structural	Fibroids, endometriosis, adenomyosis, cervical and endometrial polyps, endometrial carcinoma
Infection	Pelvic inflammatory disease (PID), STIs
Drugs	Aspirin, warfarin, chemotherapy
Systemic	Hypothyroidism, clotting disorders (Von Willebrand's disease)
Other	Intra-uterine contraceptive device (IUCD), sterilisation

Dysmenorrhoea

Dysmenorrhoea, or pain during menstruation, affects approximately 50% of menstruating women. The pain is usually a cramping lower abdominal pain that occurs several days before menstruation and usually subsides by the end of the period. The incidence of dysmenorrhoea is greatest in women in their late teens and early twenties. Primary dysmenorrhoea refers to painful periods occurring in healthy women in the absence of pathology. Secondary dysmenorrhoea is menstrual pain that is due to an underlying disease such as PID, endometriosis, adenomyosis, fibroids, adhesions and endometriosis.

Dyspareunia

The word 'dyspareunia' is derived from the Greek word *dyspareunos,* meaning 'badly mated'. It is defined as pain caused by sexual intercourse. It is broadly divided into two categories: superficial, pain during penetration felt in the introitus, and deep pain, felt with penile thrusting deep within the pelvis and against the cervix.

Causes of Superficial and Deep Dyspareunia

Superficial	Painful intercourse during penetration felt in the introitus
Psychological	Fear, ignorance, vaginismus
Infection	Candidiasis, chlamydia, trichomonas, UTI
Vaginal atrophy	Post-menopause (oestrogen deficiency), infrequent intercourse
Organic	Vaginal cancer, rectal cancer, endometriosis
Deep	Painful intercourse felt with penile thrusting deep in the pelvis
Cause	PID, cervicitis, endometriosis, adenomyosis

1.9   GYNAECOLOGY: BIMANUAL EXAMINATION

INSTRUCTIONS

You are a foundation year House Officer in general practice. Ms Okuwawa, a 35-year-old woman, has been experiencing painful heavy periods for a number of years. You have taken a history and wish to perform a bimanual examination. Perform the examination and explain to the examiner what you are doing as you proceed.

NOTE

In the OSCE setting you may be provided with a dummy instead of a real patient. Ensure that you treat it with the same courtesy and respect as you would a real patient.

INTRODUCTION

1 2 3

☐☐☐ **Introduction** — Introduce yourself. Elicit the patient's name, age and occupation. Establish rapport.

☐☐☐ **Explain** — Ensure the patient understands the nature of the examination before seeking her consent.

'I will be performing an internal examination to ensure the womb and ovaries feel healthy. This will involve introducing two gloved fingers into the vagina whilst lightly pressing on your tummy. The examination may feel a little uncomfortable but it should not be painful.'

☐☐☐ **Bladder** — Ensure the patient has emptied her bladder before proceeding. A full bladder may conceal the vagina.

☐☐☐ **Chaperone** — Inform the patient that you will ask for a chaperone.

☐☐☐ **Expose** — Ask the patient to lie flat on the couch, to take off her undergarments, bring her heels up to her bottom and allow her knees to flop apart. Expose her abdomen from the bra line to the pubic hairline. Cover her pelvic region with a towel or drape until you start the internal examination. Ensure that the patient is comfortable and maintain privacy throughout.

☐☐☐ **Abdomen** — Examine the suprapubic region and right and left iliac fossae for tenderness or masses.

BIMANUAL EXAMINATION

Gloves — Don a pair of gloves and adjust the light for maximum visibility.

☐☐☐ **Vulva** — Inspect the vulva for redness, irritation, ulceration, swellings, cyst, warts, prolapse (positive cough impulse) or any abnormal distributions of hair.

☐☐☐ **Labia** — Palpate along the length of the labia majora, feeling for any masses (cysts, carcinomas of the vulva) and palpate Bartholin's gland. Normally the gland is not palpable; however, if a non-tender mass is palpable, consider a Bartholin's cyst or a Bartholin's abscess if it is red, hot and tender.

☐☐☐ **Lubricate** — Lubricate the fingers of your gloved right hand with K-Y jelly. Part the labia with your thumb and index finger of your left hand.

☐☐☐ **Internal Exam** — Warn the patient before introducing your index and middle fingers gently into the vagina. Introduce your fingers with the palm facing medially. Gradually turn your hand through 90° so that your palm faces upwards.

Palpation — Palpate the vaginal wall, cervix, uterus and both adnexae in sequence.

Vaginal Wall — Palpate the walls of the vagina before assessing the cervix. Note any tenderness or masses.

☐☐☐ *Cervix* — Palpate the cervix with the fingertips of your right hand checking for tenderness (excitation). Comment on its size, surface, consistency and mobility.

☐☐☐ *Uterus* — Rest your left hand over the suprapubic area. Next, ballot the uterus between your two hands and attempt to catch it between the opposed fingers. Note the uterine size (enlarged – pregnancy, fibroids, endometrial carcinoma), consistency (firm, hard), mobility (immobile – endometriosis), position (retroverted, anteverted), masses (endometrial carcinoma) or tenderness.

☐☐☐ *Adnexae* — Finally, palpate the right adnexae by shifting your left hand over the right iliac fossa and internal fingers towards the right lateral fornix. Palpate the ovary and Fallopian tube (normally

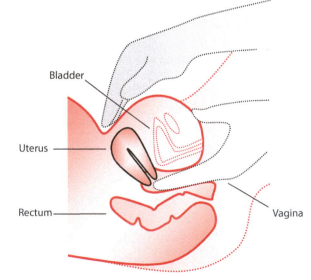

Bladder

Uterus

Rectum

Vagina

Bimanual examination

Insert two lubricated gloved fingers into the vagina. Rotate your fingers clockwise through 90 degrees. Palpate the vaginal walls, cervix, uterus and adnexae in turn. Note the uterine size, consistency, mobility, position, masses or tenderness. Feel for the adnexae by palpating between the iliac fossa and fornix. Withdraw your fingers noting any blood or discharge.

impalpable) by attempting to catch the adnexae between the fingers of both hands. Note enlarged ovaries (benign cysts, ovarian carcinoma), masses (ovarian carcinoma) or tenderness (salpingitis).

Repeat the examination on the left side, employing the same technique.

Withdrawal   Remove your fingers in same manner as they were inserted and inspect the glove for any signs of blood or discharge.

☐☐☐ **Dispose**   Throw away any remaining waste. Remove gloves and wash your hands.

Dress   Hand the patient some tissues to wipe herself, then provide her an opportunity to dress herself in privacy.

EXAMINER'S EVALUATION

1 2 3 4 5

☐☐☐☐☐   Overall assessment at performing a bimanual examination

Total mark out of 23

DIFFERENTIAL DIAGNOSIS

Fibroids

Fibroids (also known as leiomyomata) are benign tumours of the smooth muscle of the uterus (myometrium). They are the most common form of neoplasm in females, affecting 40% of all women over 40 years of age and are more common in Afro-Caribbean women. They can be single or multiple and are often round, solid, well-circumscribed nodules that vary in size from a few millimetres to large tumours that can occupy most of the abdomen. They often originate in the wall of the uterus (intramural) and may grow to bulge out of the uterus (subserosal, pedunculated) or inwards towards the cavity (submucosal, intracavitary polyps). Fibroids are oestrogen-dependent and hence increase in size during pregnancy and while the individual is on the combined pill. They reduce in size during the menopause. Patients are often asymptomatic. However, they can complain of heavy and prolonged periods (menorrhagia), dysmenorrhoea and inter-menstrual bleeding (submucosal fibroid). Submucosal fibroids can cause fertility problems including miscarriage and premature labour, whilst large fibroids can cause frequency of urinating or urinary retention due to the pressure applied on the bladder. On examination, a solid mass may be palpated that can be localised within the uterus. Multiple small fibroids may be felt as an irregular enlargement of the uterus.

Ovarian Carcinoma

Ovarian cancer is one of the most common causes of cancer-related deaths in women, commonly affecting Western women in their seventh decade of life. In its early phase it exhibits very few symptoms and is only symptomatic once it has progressed and metastasised outside the pelvis. Ovarian cancers are categorised based upon their histology, with epithelial carcinomas representing 90% of tumours. Risk factors are associated with the number of ovulations and as a result, early menarche, late menopause and nulliparous women have an increased risk whilst those with multiple pregnancies, lactation and a history of oral contraceptive use have a reduced risk. Patients who have a family history of ovarian or breast cancer have an increased risk. Ovarian carcinomas can also be familial via the BRCA1 and BRCA2 gene mutation. Symptoms include abdominal pain and distension, abnormal vaginal bleeding and changes in bowel habit. On examination, an ovarian or pelvic mass may be palpated with ascites. There may be evidence of a pleural effusion, bowel obstruction or breast symptoms due to metastasis.

Cervical Carcinoma

Cervical carcinoma is a malignant cancer of the cervix. It is the second-most common female malignancy in the UK. However, its incidence has been falling since the introduction of the cervical screening programme. Overall, 70% of malignancies are squamous carcinomas, 15% are adenocarcinomas and 15% have a mixed pattern. Risk factors include HPV, sex at a young age, multiple sexual partners, promiscuous male partners, smoking and chlamydia infection. Early stages are often asymptomatic. Symptoms of established disease include post-coital bleeding and an offensive vaginal discharge. However, inter-menstrual and post-menopausal bleeding may also be seen. Late features include an altered bowel habit, painless rectal bleeding, haematuria and chronic urinary frequency. These are suggestive of rectum, urethra and bladder involvement, respectively.

Pelvic Organ Prolapse

Pelvic organ prolapse occurs when the pelvic ligaments and the muscular floor of the pelvis become lax and weaken, causing the pelvic organs to drop. It is an umbrella term which encompasses a number of different conditions such as cystocele, urethrocele, enterocele, rectocele, uterine or vaginal vault prolapse. Symptoms often depend on the type of prolapse and can include incontinence, frequency of urination, urgency and incomplete bladder emptying (cystocele, cystourethrocele), constipation (rectocele, enterocele), impaired sexual function or heaviness or dragging sensation in the pelvic area, which patients often describe as 'my insides are falling out' (uterine prolapse). On examination, a bulge or fullness is noted in the posterior (enterocele, rectocele) or anterior (cystocele, urethrocele) vaginal wall.

Types of Pelvic Organ Prolapses

Cystocele	Bulging of the bladder into the upper two-thirds of the anterior vaginal wall
Urethrocele	Bulging of the urethra into the lower one-third of the anterior vaginal wall. Often occurs together with a prolapse of the bladder (cystourethrocele)
Enterocele	Herniation of the pouch of Douglas into the upper posterior vaginal wall. Often occurs with a rectocele or uterine prolapse
Rectocele	Prolapse of the rectum into the lower posterior vaginal wall, unlike a rectal prolapse (in which the rectum prolapses out of the anus)
Uterine	Uterus drops down into the vagina. Graded according to level of descent:
1st degree	Uterus drops slightly. Cervix remains in the vagina
2nd degree	Uterus drops further. Cervix protrudes through the introitus
3rd degree	Uterus lies entirely outside the introitus (procidentia)
Vaginal Vault	The top of the vagina (the vault) sags or bulges down into the vaginal canal. Often secondary to a hysterectomy

1.10   GYNAECOLOGY: SPECULUM EXAMINATION AND CERVICAL SMEAR TEST

INSTRUCTIONS

You are a foundation year House Officer in general practice. Ms Tanner, a 28-year-old lady, has come in for her routine smear test. Carry out the test and necessary examination, explaining to the examiner what you are doing as you proceed.

NOTE

In the OSCE setting you may be provided with a dummy instead of a real patient. Ensure that you treat it with the same courtesy and respect as you would a real patient.

INTRODUCTION

1 2 3
□□□   **Introduction**   Introduce yourself. Elicit the patient's name, age and occupation. Establish rapport.

The UK's National Cervical Cancer Screening Programme

The UK cervical cancer-screening programme was introduced in 1988 to prevent cervical cancer. Women are screened between the ages of 25 and 65 years with a 3-year interval for women aged over 25 and a 5-year interval for women aged over 50. Women aged over 65 are tested only if they have not been screened since the age of 50 or have had a recent abnormal test. Samples are taken from the squamo-columnar junction and are investigated for cervical intraepithelial neoplasms (CIN). Cellular abnormalities (dyskaryosis) are graded as mild, moderate or severe. CIN are pre-malignant cells that can develop into cervical cancer.

□□□   **Explanation**   Explain to the patient the nature of the examination before seeking consent.

'I will be performing a smear test today. This involves taking a sample from the neck of the womb, which will be checked to make sure there are no abnormalities. In order for me to take the cells, I will have to use a device known as a speculum to keep the walls of the vagina open. I will then place a brush in the opening to collect the cells from the neck of the womb, which will then be sent to the lab for investigation. The examination may feel a little uncomfortable but should not be painful.'

□□□   **Chaperone**   Inform the patient that you will obtain a chaperone.
Expose   Adequately expose the patient before examining her.

'If I may ask you to remove the clothing below your waist, lie back on the couch and cover yourself with the sheet I'll provide you with. Call me when you feel comfortable and ready to proceed.'

EQUIPMENT

- Pair of gloves
- Speculum
- Lubricant
- Pencil and investigation form
- Wooden spatula
- Slide
- Alcohol fixative spray

SMEAR TEST

☐☐☐ **Position**   Ask the patient to bring her heels towards her bottom and allow the knees to flop apart.

☐☐☐ **Prepare**   Don a pair of sterile gloves. Adjust the light for maximum visibility and choose an appropriately sized speculum. A medium-sized speculum should be appropriate for most patients, but small and large sizes are also available.

☐☐☐ **Label**   Label the vial with the patient's name, date of birth, hospital number and the date when the cervical smear was performed.

Inspection   Examine the vulva for any redness, irritation, discharge, cysts, warts or any abnormal distribution of hair.

☐☐☐ **Speculum**   Apply lubricant jelly just below the tip of the blades to avoid covering the cervix with the gel. Part the lips of the labia with your non-dominant hand. Hold the speculum so that the tip of the blade is held vertically and insert it gently into the vagina. Rotate through 90° as you progress so the handle is found anteriorly. Warn the patient before opening the blades. Opening the blades will stretch the wall of the vagina, bringing the cervix into view. Lock the blades into position by tightening the screw once the cervix is visualised.

☐☐☐ **Sample Cells**   Introduce the brush to the external os and then gently rotate. Remove the brush and insert into the vial. Snap off the head and close the vial firmly.

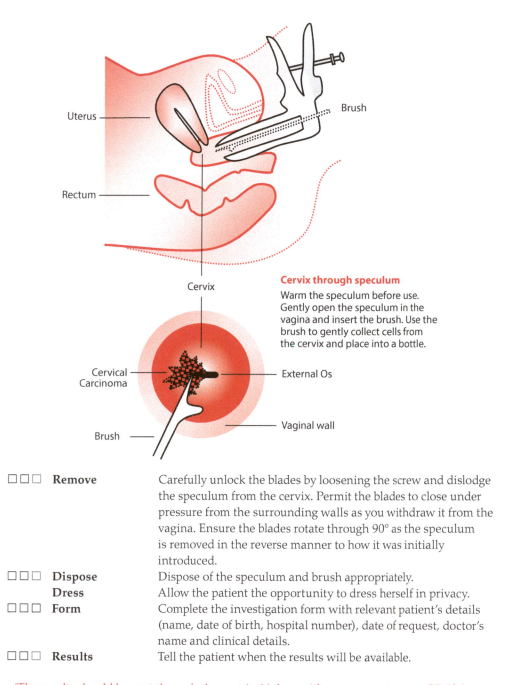

Uterus

Rectum

Brush

Cervix

Cervix through speculum

Warm the speculum before use. Gently open the speculum in the vagina and insert the brush. Use the brush to gently collect cells from the cervix and place into a bottle.

Cervical Carcinoma

External Os

Brush

Vaginal wall

☐☐☐ **Remove** Carefully unlock the blades by loosening the screw and dislodge the speculum from the cervix. Permit the blades to close under pressure from the surrounding walls as you withdraw it from the vagina. Ensure the blades rotate through 90° as the speculum is removed in the reverse manner to how it was initially introduced.

☐☐☐ **Dispose** Dispose of the speculum and brush appropriately.

Dress Allow the patient the opportunity to dress herself in privacy.

☐☐☐ **Form** Complete the investigation form with relevant patient's details (name, date of birth, hospital number), date of request, doctor's name and clinical details.

☐☐☐ **Results** Tell the patient when the results will be available.

'The results should be sent through the post in 14 days with a copy sent to your GP. If the results are negative then the cells are healthy and we will see you again for routine check in 3 years' time. If the cervical smear is not negative it may need to be interpreted and explained by your GP. On occasion an inadequate sample may have been taken, which means that you may have to repeat the test.'

Management of Abnormal Cervical Smears

Result	Management
Negative	Inform patient and repeat after 3 years (> 25 yr) or 5 years (> 50 yr)
Inadequate	Repeat the test within 3 months. If three consecutive inadequate samples are collected, refer for colposcopy
Borderline/Mild dyskaryosis	Samples are then tested for Human Papilloma Virus (HPV) DNA
	HPV negative – return to routine screening
	HPV inadequate/equivocal – repeat smear and HPV in six months' time
	HPV positive – refer for colposcopy (NHS England Guidance)
Moderate dyskaryosis	Refer for colposcopy
Severe dyskaryosis	Refer urgently for colposcopy

Complications   Inform the patient that she may experience some spotting for a day or two after the examination but it should not be heavy or painful.

Using a Cervex-Brush and Liquid-Based Cytology (LBC) Vial

The Cervex-Brush broom is a soft, pyramid-shaped brush that allows the simultaneous collection of ectocervical, endocervical and transformation zone cells in a single sample. It is significantly more efficient than the previous wooden spatula technique in obtaining adequate cervical smears and ensuring fewer repeat smears. Numerous studies have showed that liquid-based cytology is more sensitive than previous smear cytology.

To collect a cell sample, introduce the broom into the canal approximately 2 cm in length, similar to the length of the brush. Allow the central bristles to lie within the endocervical canal while the outer bristles rest against the ectocervix. Rotate the brush clockwise through only five cycles before removing it from the canal. Next check the expiry date of the liquid-based cytology vial. Apply gentle pressure against the back of the brush head, allowing it to snap off from the main stem and rest inside the preservative vial. Further samples can be placed into the same vial and must be documented in the request form. Apply the cap to the vial and tighten. Document the patient's name, date of birth and date of sample on the vial.

EXAMINER'S EVALUATION

1 2 3 4 5
☐ ☐ ☐ ☐ ☐   Overall assessment on performing a smear test
Total mark out of 20

INSTRUCTIONS

You are a foundation year House Officer in obstetrics. Mrs Gandhi has grade 3 placenta praevia and has been admitted for elective Caesarean section at 36 weeks. You have been assigned the task of inserting a pre-op urinary catheter. Explain to the patient what you will do and insert the catheter with the equipment provided. Explain to the examiner what you are doing as you proceed.

INTRODUCTION

1 2 3

☐☐☐ **Introduction**   Introduce yourself. Elicit the patient's name, age and occupation. Establish rapport.

☐☐☐ **Explain**   Ensure that the patient understands the nature of the examination before seeking consent.

'As you will be having a Caesarean section we will need to monitor the amount of urine that you will be producing during the procedure. I will therefore have to insert a urinary catheter. This is a simple procedure that involves inserting a small flexible plastic tube through your water pipe and into your bladder. It should not be painful, but may feel a little uncomfortable. Do you have any questions or concerns?'

          Consent   Obtain consent before beginning the procedure.

☐☐☐ **Chaperone**   Inform the patient that you will ask for a chaperone.

          Equipment   Collect and set up the equipment and place it on the bottom shelf of trolley.

EQUIPMENT

- Catheterisation pack
- Catheter bag
- Sterile gloves
- Lignocaine gel (Instilagel prefilled)
- Three plastic prongs
- Foley catheter 12 or 14
- Antiseptic solution (chlorhexidine)
- Adhesive tape
- 10 mL syringe (+1 green needle)
- 10 mL sterile water

PROCEDURE

*Trolley

☐☐☐ **Preparation**
Put on an apron, clean the trolley using bactericidal spray and wash hands.

☐☐☐ **Expose**
Ask the patient to lie flat on the couch and to take off her undergarments and bring her heels up to her bottom. Maintain the patient's dignity by covering her with a sheet. Ensure that the patient is comfortable and maintain privacy throughout.

☐☐☐ **Sterile Field**
Peel the outer plastic covering of the catheterisation pack and slide the pack onto the trolley. Unwrap the paper covering, touching only the outside of the paper, and form a sterile area. Stick the yellow disposable bag onto the side of the trolley. Place the above equipment in a sterile manner into the area. Check the expiry date of the chlorhexidine solution and then pour it into a small pot with swabs (found in catheter pack). Open a 10 mL vial of sterile water and then place it outside the sterile field.

☐☐☐ **Gloves**
Don a pair of sterile gloves.

Preparation
Squeeze a small amount of lignocaine gel into the cardboard receptacle. Take the 10 mL syringe and attach the green needle to draw up the sterile water. Dip the needle into the vial (outside the sterile field) without touching it (or ask assistance). After drawing up 10 mL, dispose of the needle in the sharps bin and replace the syringe in the sterile field. Finally, remove the tip of the end of the catheter sheath.

*Patient

☐☐☐ **Drape and Gauze**
Make a hole in the drape and place it appropriately over the patient to maintain a sterile field.

☐☐☐ **Clean Labia**
Holding a wet chlorhexidine-soaked swab with a plastic prong, wipe the right labia minor only. Dispose of the swab and prong. Taking a newly soaked swab and prong, cleanse the left labia minor once only, then dispose of this swab and prong. Finally, separate the labia with your left hand using a piece of gauze, take a new wet swab and prong and clean the urethral meatus with your right hand. Dispose of the swab as before.

If there has been any contact between the gloves and the non-sterile area while cleaning, it is important to put on a second pair of sterile gloves before inserting the catheter.

*Catheter

☐☐☐ **Preparation**
Place the catheter (still in its plastic covering), into the cardboard receptacle and put it between the patient's legs.

Lignocaine
Massage the end of the catheter out by a few centimetres. Dip the tip of the catheter into the LA jelly previously deposited in the receptacle.

☐☐☐   **Insert Catheter**   Hold the labia open with one hand and introduce the catheter tip, via its sleeve, into the urethral orifice by approximately 5–6 cm. Keep the end of the catheter over the receptacle to catch any sudden flow of urine. Once urine starts to flow, advance the catheter a further 1–2 cm to ensure the balloon is in the bladder.

☐☐☐   **Inflate Balloon**   Inflate the catheter balloon with 1 mL of sterile water. Ask the patient to say if she feels any pain. Continue filling slowly with the remaining 9 mL, asking patient if she is in any pain, and observe the patient's face for grimacing as you inflate the balloon. Gently tug on the catheter to make sure that the balloon becomes lodged in the neck of the bladder.

☐☐☐   **Catheter Bag**   Attach the drainage bag to the end of the catheter and tape the catheter to the thigh.

☐☐☐   **Dispose**   Dispose of waste appropriately.

☐☐☐   **Document**   Document in the notes the size of catheter used and the residual volume of urine initially collected.

EXAMINER'S EVALUATION

1 2 3 4 5
☐ ☐ ☐ ☐ ☐   Overall assessment of inserting female catheter
Total mark out of 23

1.12   GYNAECOLOGY: OVARIAN CYST

INSTRUCTIONS

You are a foundation year House Officer in a gynaecology outpatient clinic. Ms Atkin is a 29-year-old woman who has been referred to the clinic by her GP following a routine PV examination. The ultrasound scan demonstrated a 6.5 cm fluid-filled sac with regular borders on her right ovary. Explain these findings to the patient and tell her what will happen next.

HISTORY

1 2 3

□□□ **Introduction**   Introduce yourself. Elicit her name, age and occupation. Establish rapport.

      History   Take a brief history of her presenting complaint, including pain, irregular periods, nausea and vomiting.

□□□ **Ideas**   Ask the patient if she has any ideas of what may be causing her symptoms.

□□□ **Concerns**   Ask the patient if she has any worries or concerns about her symptoms.

Ovarian Cyst

Symptoms, Signs and Investigation Findings

Ovarian cysts are usually asymptomatic and are often discovered as an incidental finding on a pelvic ultrasound scan. If they are symptomatic they may present with irregular menses or vaginal spotting and produce symptoms secondary to a mass effect. They are found in nearly all premenopausal women, and in up to 15% of postmenopausal women. They can affect women at any age but are more common in women of childbearing age. Functional cysts are by far the most common type and include follicular cysts and corpus luteal cysts. Follicular cysts occur in the first two weeks of the cycle when the ovarian follicle fails to rupture and release an egg but instead continues to grow. When it does rupture it causes a sudden-onset, sharp, severe, unilateral pain, typically during mid-cycle (*mittelschmerz*). Luteal cysts represent failed degeneration of the corpus luteum and tend to produce symptoms when they become inflamed or haemorrhage spontaneously, often in the later half of the cycle. Others include theca lutein cysts (due to high HCG levels) and chocolate cysts (blood-filled cysts that are frequently painful). On ultrasound investigation, unilateral cystic lesions < 10 cm in diameter with regular borders are most likely to be benign. Lesions that persist beyond 2 months and are > 10 cm in diameter with irregular borders or thick septa should be investigated for possible malignancy.

MEDICAL ADVICE

☐☐☐ **Ultrasound**   Break the news empathetically, using pauses where appropriate. The information should be paced with good use of body language and silence.

'I have the results of your ultrasound scan. It shows there is a medium-sized fluid sac within your right ovary. This is known an ovarian cyst. Have you ever been told that you have an ovarian cyst and can you tell me what you understand by it?'

☐☐☐ **Ovarian Cyst**   Explain the diagnosis in simple terms the patient understands.

'Ovarian cysts are fluid-filled sacs located in the ovaries of women. They are quite common and most of them are quite harmless. During a woman's normal cycle, small cysts develop in the ovaries and usually disappear before the next cycle. Sometimes, for various reasons, your hormones may become unbalanced and, instead of disappearing, these cysts grow in size. Usually they are quite harmless and disappear within 6 weeks. On very rare occasions they can turn out to be cancerous.'

☐☐☐ **Observe**   Explain to the patient that a repeat US will be performed in 4 weeks' time.

'In most cases we normally watch and wait to see what will happen with the cyst. We will repeat an ultrasound in 4 weeks' time to see if the cyst has shrunk in size.'

☐☐☐ **Surgery**   Explain to the patient when surgery may be indicated.

'If you are suffering from symptoms due to the ovarian cyst such as severe pain, fever and vomiting, or if the cyst is exceptionally large, then we would advise that the cyst should be removed surgically.

'We will need to keep you in hospital and perform the surgery to drain the cyst. This will be done laparoscopically, which is otherwise known as keyhole surgery. You will be put to sleep and the surgeon will make two small incisions in your tummy. The cyst will be drained and a small sample removed and sent to the laboratory. In exceptional cases, open surgery may have to be carried out if keyhole surgery fails.'

☐☐☐ **Symptoms**   Advise the patient when to seek medical help.

'Although generally cysts do not cause any symptoms, you should seek medical help if you begin to suffer from the following: pain with fever and vomiting, sudden severe abdominal pain, faintness or dizziness.'

☐☐☐ **Recurrence** Explain to the patient what treatments are available in case of recurrence.

'If you suffer from recurrent ovarian cysts, some treatments are available such as the combined oral contraceptive or the depot contraceptive injections that can reduce the rate of recurrence. You can discuss this further with your GP if the need arises.'

Summarise Summarise back to the patient what you have explained so far.

CLOSING

☐☐☐ **Understanding** Confirm that the patient has understood what you have explained to her.

☐☐☐ **Questions** Respond appropriately to the patient's questions.
Leaflet Offer to give her more information in the form of a handout. Advise that the leaflet contains much of the information you have mentioned.

COMMUNICATION SKILLS

☐☐☐ **Rapport** Attempt to establish rapport with the patient through the use of appropriate eye contact. Maintain appropriate body language and an open posture throughout.

☐☐☐ **Listening** Demonstrate an interest and concern in what the patient says. Show active listening and listen empathetically.

☐☐☐ **Empathy** Demonstrate an empathetic response (offer emotional support and validate concerns).

EXAMINER'S EVALUATION

1 2 3 4 5
☐☐☐☐☐ Overall assessment of explaining ovarian cysts
☐☐☐☐☐ Role player's score
Total mark out of 27

1.13   GYNAECOLOGY: MISCARRIAGE

INSTRUCTIONS

You are a foundation year House Officer in A&E where you have seen to Mrs Nikalou, a nulliparous 24-year-old woman 12 weeks into her first pregnancy. She is very anxious and has noticed blood on her underwear. The ultrasound shows a gestational sac of 70 mm and crown–rump length of 60 mm. No foetal heart sounds were heard. Explain the results to the patient and what will need to be done next.

HISTORY

1 2 3

☐☐☐	**Introduction**	Introduce yourself. Elicit the patient's name, age and occupation. Establish rapport.
	History	Take a brief history of the presenting complaint, including when the bleeding started, how much and any associated symptoms, i.e. pain.
☐☐☐	**Ideas**	Ask the patient if she has any idea what may be causing her symptoms.
☐☐☐	**Concerns**	Ask the patient if she has any worries or concerns about her symptoms.

Miscarriages

Symptoms, Signs and Ultrasonic Findings

A miscarriage or spontaneous abortion is defined as the loss of a foetus before 20 weeks of gestation. Up to 20% of all pregnancies miscarry, with 80% occurring in first trimester. The frequency of miscarriage decreases with increasing gestational age. Symptoms include a history of vaginal bleeding with blood clots and severe suprapubic abdominal pain. The vaginal bleeding may be significant enough to soak tampons, pads, sanitary towels or even clothes. Contractions and abdominal pain may co-exist but tend to resolve in a complete abortion. This is associated with the passage of products of conception and a cessation of vaginal bleeding. An ultrasound scan is the investigation of choice for suspected cases of miscarriages. Ultrasonic features consistent with a non-viable pregnancy include:

- An embryo with absent heartbeat when the CRL is >5 mm
- Loss of previously observed foetal cardiac activity
- Irregular-edged or collapsed gestational sac
- Abnormal echogenic material within the uterine cavity
- Lack of growth of the sac or foetal pole over a 5-day period

Foetal heart sounds are good markers for a viable pregnancy, with the risk of spontaneous abortion decreasing from 50% to 3%. The earliest time they can be detected is by week 5 of gestation or when the crown-rump length is 2 to 4 mm and the gestational sac is 10 mm.

*Breaking Bad News

☐☐☐ **Ultrasound**   Break the bad news empathetically, using pauses where appropriate. Pace the information and ensure that you use appropriate body language and silence.

'I have the results of your ultrasound. Unfortunately, I have to break some difficult news to you. I am afraid it is more serious than we had expected. Your scan suggests that the baby has stopped growing and I am sorry to have to tell you that you are having a miscarriage.'

MEDICAL ADVICE

☐☐☐ **Miscarriage**   Explain the diagnosis in simple terms the patient understands.

'Firstly, I would like you to know that this is not your fault. Miscarriages occur in about 20% of pregnancies and in most cases it is due to a random event. There is nothing you could have done to prevent it.'

*What Will Happen Next

☐☐☐ **Options**   Explain to the patient the available options in relation to her miscarriage. Take care to be sensitive and acknowledge her emotions.

Conservative

'Most women will cope with a miscarriage naturally without any need for us to do anything. This usually takes place over a week. However, if after a week you do not think that you have come to terms with the loss of the pregnancy or if you are still having heavy and painful bleeding, please return to see the gynaecological specialist.'

ERPC

'If you have been bleeding a lot, or if some of the pregnancy still remains in your womb, you may require a simple procedure to help remove it. This is known as an evacuation of retained products of conception (ERPC). This is a simple operation which should only last up to 15 minutes and you will be asleep during it.'

☐☐☐ **Rhesus**   Explain to the patient the need to check her Rhesus status.

'I now need to take some blood from you to check your Rhesus status. This is to determine if there may be a slight reaction between the baby's blood and yours. This reaction will not cause any problems now but may affect future pregnancies. If there is a problem then you may need an injection to prevent any harm in future pregnancies.'

☐☐☐   **Discharge**   Explain to the patient what will happen after discharge.

'On returning home you may continue to bleed for up to 10 days, but the bleeding should not be heavy or painful. Use sanitary towels until the bleeding has stopped and avoid sexual intercourse. You may experience period-like pains, for which you can take simple painkillers. Expect your next period to start within 6 weeks and you can return to work when you feel ready. If you require a medical sick note, we can facilitate this.'

☐☐☐   **Follow-up**   Offer the patient details of support groups and follow-up.

'Having a miscarriage can be a very emotional and lonely time for you. If you feel that you need to talk to someone we can put you in touch with a support group called the Miscarriage Association. This group consists of women who have all experienced miscarriages and will be able to answer any questions or anxieties you may have.'

☐☐☐   **Summarise**   Summarise back to the patient what you have explained so far.

CLOSING

☐☐☐   **Understanding**   Confirm that the patient has understood what you have
                             explained to her.
☐☐☐   **Questions**   Respond appropriately to the patient's questions.
☐☐☐   **Leaflet**   Offer to give her more information in the form of a handout.
                             Advise her that the leaflet contains much of the information you
                             have mentioned.

COMMUNICATION SKILLS

☐☐☐   **Rapport**   Attempt to establish rapport with the patient through the use
                             of appropriate eye contact. Maintain appropriate body language
                             and an open posture throughout.
☐☐☐   **Listening**   Demonstrate interest and concern in what the patient says. Show
                             active listening and listen empathetically.
☐☐☐   **Pauses**   Pace the information and use appropriate pauses. Allow the
                             patient to speak her feelings freely and without interruption.
☐☐☐   **Empathy**   Respond empathetically (offer emotional support and validate
                             her concerns).
☐☐☐   **Verbal Cues**   Use non-verbal and verbal cues, i.e. tone and pace of voice, and
                             nod head where appropriate.

EXAMINER'S EVALUATION

1 2 3 4 5
☐☐☐☐☐   Overall assessment of miscarriage counselling
☐☐☐☐☐   Role player's score
         Total mark out of 31

1.14   GYNAECOLOGY: ABORTION

INSTRUCTIONS

You are a foundation year House Officer in general practice. Ms Goldsberg, a 21-year-old woman, has done a pregnancy test that has shown that she is pregnant. Her last menstrual period was 7 weeks ago. She is very distressed when you see her today. Elicit her needs and give her appropriate advice and further management options.

HISTORY

1 2 3

☐☐☐ **Introduction**   Introduce yourself. Elicit her name, age and occupation. Establish rapport.

'I understand that your recent pregnancy test was positive and you are feeling quite distressed about this. I am sorry that you are feeling this way. Can you tell me more about this?'

☐☐☐ **Ideas**   Explore her ideas regarding the pregnancy and what she wants to achieve.

'I can see that this is very difficult for you right now. Have you had any ideas or thoughts of whether you would like to keep this pregnancy?'

☐☐☐ **Concerns**   Elicit the concerns the patient has about keeping the pregnancy (its legality, its effect on any future pregnancy).

'I understand that you are considering an abortion. Do you have any particular worries or concerns about this? Have you given this decision much thought? Do you wish to speak to someone before you make a decision?'

☐☐☐ **Sexual History**   Take a brief sexual history including her current relationship, her consent to intercourse, her use of any contraception and contraception failure (condom split). Also enquire about previous pregnancies or terminations.

☐☐☐ **Menstrual History** Elicit the patient's last menstrual period (LMP). Enquire about the length and regularity of her cycles.

Social History   Enquire about her home situation, including who lives at home, whether she has discussed her decision with her partner and if she wants to include anyone else in the decision-making process.

MEDICAL ADVICE

☐☐☐ **Legality**   Explain to the patient that abortions are legal before a pregnancy age of 24 weeks.

'I wish to reassure you that as you are only 7 weeks pregnant it is perfectly legal for you to have an abortion, since in the UK the legal cut-off point is 24 weeks.'

The UK's Abortion Law

The UK Abortion Act of 1967

Termination of pregnancy was legalised in the UK under the 1967 Abortion Act. It can be artificially induced up to 24 weeks of pregnancy. In the UK 90% of abortions take place before 12 weeks. Two doctors (e.g. the GP and a gynaecologist) must give their consent, stating that to continue with the pregnancy would:

- endanger the life of the mother
- endanger the physical or mental health of the mother
- be a risk to the physical or mental health of the siblings
- risk that the foetus would be born handicapped.

Most abortions in the UK fall under the second category. Patients must be referred for a termination of pregnancy by their GP, family planning centre or private health centre. No doctor is obliged to consent to or participate in an abortion, but all have a duty of care to refer the individual to the correct department. The 1967 Abortion Act does not extend to Northern Ireland, where abortion is still illegal.

	Accessibility	State that the service is free under the National Health Service.
☐☐☐	**Confidentiality**	Reassure the patient that the procedure will remain confidential.
	Appointments	Explain that she will be given two separate appointments. The first is to assess eligibility and choice of procedure; the second will be the procedure itself. Also mention that the abortion should be completed within 3 weeks of the first contact she has made with the services.
☐☐☐	**Options**	Explain the options available to the patient for the termination of her pregnancy.

Option 1

'I understand that you wish to proceed with the abortion. I would like to explain the different options available. The first option is to abort the pregnancy using tablets. You will be given a tablet called mifepristone, which stops the pregnancy hormones from working and makes you have an early miscarriage. A few days after this you will be given another tablet that can be taken by mouth or inserted into the vagina, which will cause the pregnancy to be expelled. This option is 99% successful if used before 8 weeks and must be carried out before the pregnancy has reached 9 weeks.'

Option 2

'The second option is a minor surgical procedure which is usually performed before the pregnancy has reached its 15th week. You will not need to be put to sleep since it will be done under local anaesthetic. A small tube will be passed into the womb and the pregnancy will be removed. This is a fairly quick procedure and should only take 5 minutes.'

Option 3

'After 15 weeks of pregnancy, a more extensive surgical procedure is required. This involves putting you to sleep under general anaesthetic and removing the pregnancy through a tube passed into your womb. You may need to stay overnight in the hospital after the procedure has been carried out.'

☐☐☐ **Complications** Explain to the patient potential complications when undertaking a termination of pregnancy, such as infection, heavy bleeding, potential damage to the cervix or womb, minimal chance of affecting fertility and a failure to terminate the pregnancy, requiring further treatment.

☐☐☐ **Rhesus Status** Explain to the patient the need to check their Rhesus status and that, if necessary, anti-D injection may need to be administered.

☐☐☐ **Screen STDs** Explain to the patient that all women attending for an abortion are screened for chlamydia to reduce the chances of post-operation infection (salpingitis).

☐☐☐ **Implications** Discuss with the patient possible implications after having the abortion, such as her fertility not being compromised and possible emotional response.

Fertility

'It is important to appreciate that having a successful abortion will not compromise your future chances of falling pregnant.'

Counsellor

'After having an abortion, some women experience a number of different emotions. You may feel relieved or sad. All of this is perfectly natural. If you are having problems coping with your emotions, I can put you in touch with a counsellor, if you feel you need to talk to someone.'

☐☐☐ **Contraception** Discuss with the patient available contraceptive options.
    Summarise Summarise back to the patient what you have explained so far.

CLOSING

☐☐☐ **Understanding**   Confirm that the patient has understood what you have explained to her.

☐☐☐ **Questions**   Respond appropriately to the patient's questions.
Leaflet   Offer to give her more information in the form of a handout. Advise that the leaflet contains much of the information you have mentioned.

COMMUNICATION SKILLS

☐☐☐ **Rapport**   Attempt to establish rapport with the patient through the use of appropriate eye contact. Maintain appropriate body language and an open posture throughout.

☐☐☐ **Listening**   Demonstrate interest and concern in what the patient says. Show active listening and listen empathetically.

☐☐☐ **Pauses**   Pace the information and use appropriate pauses. Allow the patient to speak her feelings freely and without interruption.

☐☐☐ **Empathy**   Demonstrate an empathetic response (offer emotional support and validate the patient's concerns).

☐☐☐ **Verbal Cues**   Use non-verbal and verbal cues, i.e. tone and pace of voice, nod head where appropriate.

EXAMINER'S EVALUATION

1 2 3 4 5
☐☐☐☐☐ Overall assessment of abortion counselling
☐☐☐☐☐ Role player's score
Total mark out of 33

1.15 GYNAECOLOGY: ECTOPIC PREGNANCY

INSTRUCTIONS

You are a foundation year House Officer in obstetrics. An 18-year-old woman presents with colicky right iliac fossa pain. She mentions that she has had vaginal bleeding the last 3 days and missed her period 2 months prior. Her pregnancy test is positive and an urgent ultrasound performed by your registrar fails to demonstrate an intra-uterine pregnancy. Explain the likely diagnosis and next course of action.

HISTORY

1 2 3

☐☐☐ **Introduction**   Introduce yourself. Elicit the patient's name, age and occupation. Establish rapport.

☐☐☐ **History**   Take a brief history of the presenting complaint, including when the pain started, its location and associated symptoms, i.e. vaginal bleeding, vomiting, fever.

☐☐☐ **Ideas**   Ask the patient if she has any ideas of what may be causing her symptoms.

☐☐☐ **Concerns**   Ask the patient if she has any worries or concerns about her symptoms.

Ectopic Pregnancy

Symptoms, Signs and Investigation Findings

Ectopic pregnancy is defined as the implantation of an embryo outside of the uterine cavity. It complicates 1% of all pregnancies and represents a major cause of maternal mortality. The most common site for implantation is the inside lining of a Fallopian tube (97%). Other sites include the cornu, cervix, ovary and peritoneum. Ectopic pregnancy should always be suspected in a sexually active woman who presents with bleeding or abdominal pain. Clinical features include a 4–10 week history of amenorrhoea, sudden onset of colicky lower abdominal pain (later becoming constant) and scanty dark vaginal bleeding. Intraperitoneal haemorrhage is heralded by syncopal collapse and shoulder tip pain. The diagnosis is suggested by an empty uterus on ultrasound with a positive pregnancy test (beta-HCG levels). A confirmed diagnosis is characterised by the presence of a thick, ring-like echogenic centre located outside the uterus, with a gestational sac containing a foetal pole or yolk sac.

---

*Breaking Bad News

☐☐☐   **Ultrasound**   Break the bad news empathetically, using pauses where appropriate. The information should be paced with a good use of body language and silence.

'I have the results of your ultrasound. Unfortunately, I have to break some difficult news to you. I am afraid it is more serious than we thought. Your scan suggests that the pregnancy is growing outside your womb. This is known as an ectopic pregnancy. The most common place for it to occur is in your Fallopian tubes and this may the reason why you are suffering from pain and bleeding. I'm sorry to have to tell you that your pregnancy is not viable and will have to be removed for your own safety.'

MEDICAL ADVICE

☐☐☐   **Ectopic Preg.**   Explain the diagnosis to the patient in simple terms the patient understands.

'Firstly, I would like you to know that this is not your fault and there was nothing that you could have done to prevent this. Ectopic pregnancies can occur for a number of different reasons, such as suffering from infection or inflammation of the tubes, previous surgery and a condition known as endometriosis. However, in most causes no cause is found.'

☐☐☐   **Surgery**   Explain to the patient why a surgical procedure needs to be undertaken in order to remove the pregnancy.

'As we mentioned before, it is likely that the pregnancy is in one of your tubes and not in the womb. Your tubes were not designed to stretch or grow the way your womb would and are at risk of rupturing if the pregnancy continues. For this reason, we will have to remove the pregnancy and maybe your tube as well. It is important to appreciate that if we do not do this, your Fallopian tube may burst, putting your life at serious risk.'

☐☐☐   **Laparoscopy**   Explain to the patient the laparoscopic procedure.

'We will need to keep you in hospital and perform surgery to remove the pregnancy from your tubes. This will be done laparoscopically, which is otherwise known as keyhole surgery. You will be put to sleep and the surgeon will make two small incisions in your tummy. The pregnancy will be identified and removed, making all attempts to leave your tubes intact. In exceptional cases, open surgery may have to be carried out if the keyhole surgery fails.'

☐☐☐   **Alternatives**   Explain alternative methods of managing the ectopic pregnancy.

'In most cases we undertake keyhole surgery to remove the ectopic pregnancy. However, in a minority of cases and depending on your circumstances, there are two alternative options which may be indicated. The first is simply watching and waiting. In some situations the pregnancy stops growing by itself and disappears without consequence. However, you must be fit and well and blood tests for your pregnancy hormone levels should show a drop before this option can be fully considered.

'The second option is to give an injection called methotrexate. This will cause the pregnancy to stop and shrink away. However, we consider this only in women whose pregnancy hormone levels are already very low.'

☐☐☐ **Advice**   Explain to the patient the increased risk of future ectopic pregnancies.

'Normally, we advise women to wait for three normal periods before trying to fall pregnant again. I must inform you that since you have had an ectopic pregnancy you have a small but significant risk of it occurring again (10%). Therefore, we advise you to visit your GP following a positive pregnancy test so that you can have an early ultrasound scan to make sure the pregnancy is in the womb.'

CLOSING

☐☐☐ **Follow-up** Offer the patient details of support groups and follow-up.

'Having an ectopic pregnancy can be very emotionally draining. If you feel that you need to talk to someone about how you are feeling, we can give you details of some support groups and, if need be, we can get you to speak to a counsellor if you would like.'

☐☐☐ **Understanding** Confirm that the patient has understood what you have explained to her.

☐☐☐ **Questions** Respond appropriately to the patient's questions.

   Leaflet   Offer to give her more information in the form of a handout. Advise that the leaflet contains much of the information you have mentioned.

   Summarise Summarise back to the patient what you have explained so far.

COMMUNICATION SKILLS

☐☐☐ **Rapport**   Attempt to establish rapport with the patient through the use of appropriate eye contact. Maintain appropriate body language and an open posture throughout.

☐☐☐ **Listening** Demonstrate interest and concern in what the patient says. Show active listening and listen empathetically.

☐☐☐ **Pauses**   Pace the information and use appropriate pauses. Allow the patient to speak her feelings freely and without interruption.

☐☐☐ **Empathy** Demonstrate an empathetic response (offer emotional support and validate her concerns).

☐☐☐ **Verbal Cues** Use non-verbal and verbal cues, i.e. tone and pace of voice, and nod head where appropriate.

EXAMINER'S EVALUATION

1 2 3 4 5

☐ ☐ ☐ ☐ ☐   Overall assessment of explaining ectopic pregnancy

☐ ☐ ☐ ☐ ☐   Role player's score

Total mark out of 31

Sexual Health

2

2.1   SEXUAL HEALTH: SEXUAL HISTORY

INSTRUCTIONS

You are a foundation year House Officer in a GUM clinic. Ms Franklin has presented with a vaginal discharge. Take a full sexual history from the patient. Elicit her concerns and answer any questions she may have. You will be marked on your ability to elicit a sexual history.

INTRODUCTION

1 2 3

☐☐☐ **Introduction**   Introduce yourself. Elicit the patient's name and age. Establish rapport.

'I would like to ask you some personal questions about your sex life. It is OK if you prefer not to answer some of them. I just want to reassure you that any information you do give me will be treated in the strictest confidence.'

☐☐☐ **Occupation**   Enquire about the patient's present occupation.

HISTORY

☐☐☐ **Concerns**   Elicit all the patient's presenting concerns. Use open questions and explore the patient's beliefs about their health. For each concern or complaint, elicit the patient's ideas, concerns and expectations.

☐☐☐ **History**   For each complaint ascertain the time of onset, presenting features and associated symptoms. Explore each symptom systematically.

☐☐☐ **Discharge**   'Have you noticed any discharge? Where have you noticed it (in the vagina, urethra, under foreskin, anal)? How long have you had it for? What colour is it? Does it smell (fishy)? Is it itchy?'

Different Colours of Discharge

Clear/white	Physiological (increased in pregnancy, puberty, OCP)
White/yellow	Atrophic vaginitis (dyspareunia, soreness, light bleeding), chlamydia (discharge rare, dysuria)
White/grey	Bacterial vaginosis (fishy odour, no itchiness, dysuria, pH > 4.5)
Cottage cheese	Candidiasis (redness, itchiness, dysuria, pH < 4.5)
Green/grey	Trichomonas (frothy, odour, dyspareunia, itch, inflamed cervix, pH > 4.5)
Green/yellow	Gonorrhoea (odour, dysuria)
Red/brown	Cervical/endometrial carcinoma (foul-smelling, weight loss)

☐☐☐ **Urinary Sympt.**   'Do you get any burning or pain when passing urine (dysuria)? Are you passing urine more often (frequency)? Are you waking

☐☐☐ **Pain**
up at night to pass urine (nocturia)? Do you feel that when you want to go to the toilet you must go there and then (urgency)?'
'Do you have any abdominal pain (male – penile, testicular)? When did it first start? Is it sharp or dull in nature?'

☐☐☐ **Symptoms**
'Have you noticed any fevers itchiness, rashes, pain during intercourse (dyspareunia) or joint pains?'

SEXUAL HISTORY

☐☐☐ **Active**
'Are you currently sexually active or have you been active in the last 3 months?'

☐☐☐ **Contacts**
'Do you have a regular or casual partner? Male or female? When was the last time you had sex? Currently how many partners do you have? Have they experienced similar symptoms?'

☐☐☐ **Type**
'Have you practised vaginal sex? Did you use protection? What type did you use (condoms, oral contraceptive pill, diaphragm)? Did you practice oral or anal sex? Did you give it or receive it? Did you use protection?'

☐☐☐ **Location**
'Have you had sex abroad? Where is your partner from? Do you know if your partner has had a sexual partner from Africa or East Asia?'

☐☐☐ **STDs and HIV**
'Have you or your partner ever had a sexually transmitted disease, such as chlamydia, gonorrhoea or syphilis? Was it successfully treated? Have you or your partner ever had an HIV test?'

ASSOCIATED HISTORY

☐☐☐ **Menstrual Hist.**
'When was your last period (LMP)? How long do your cycles last? Are your cycles regular? Do you have any pain or bleeding?'

Obstetric Hist.
'Do you have any children? How many? What type of delivery did they have? Have you had any miscarriages or terminations?'

☐☐☐ **Gynae. History**
'Have you had a smear test? Was it normal?'

Medical History
'Do you suffer from any medical illness? Have you ever been admitted to hospital?'

☐☐☐ **Drug History**
'Do you take any medications? Are you on any oral contraceptive pills?'

Social History
'Do you smoke? Do you drink alcohol? Do you take recreational drugs?'

CLOSING

☐☐☐ **Follow-up**
Say that you would like to perform an examination and take a high vaginal swab (HVS) for culturing. Suggest that you wish to check for chlamydia, gonorrhoea and syphilis.

☐☐☐ **Contact Tracing**
Explain to the patient the importance of testing their partners and provide a contact slip.

Disease	Symptoms	Risk factors	Signs
Candidiasis (thrush)	Commonest cause of vaginitis, 20% asymptomatic, cheesy white discharge, pruritus – superficial dyspareunia and dysuria	Pregnancy, diabetes, recent antibiotics, hospital stay	Vulval redness and irritation Men: red, irritable, patchy sores on the foreskin and glans
Bacterial vaginosis (Gardnerella vaginalis)	Not STD. Greyish white discharge with fishy odour – worse after sex. Not itchy. 50% asymptomatic	IUD in situ.	Discharge only usual sign.
Chlamydia – women (Chlamydia trachomatis)	75% asymptomatic – sexual transmission. Chronic: chronic pelvic pain, dyspareunia, inter-menstrual bleeding. Can lead to pelvic inflammatory disease.	Sexually active, age < 25, occasionally vertical transmission, recent change in sexual partner	Initial signs: yellow discharge and ureteritis. Chronic: intermenstrual bleeding Reiter's syndrome: arthritis, conjunctivitis, ureteritis. Fitz-Hugh–Curtis syndrome – inflammation of Glisson's capsule – gonorrhaea assoc. or chlamydia.
Chlamydia – men (Chlamydia trachomatis)	50% asymptomatic ureteritis, mild discharge, testicular pain	As above Anal sex	Epidydmo-orchitis Rare (non-gender specific) – ocular trachoma Proctitis – rectal infection Lymphogranuloma venereum.
Gonorrhoea (female) Neisseria gonorrhoeae	50% women asymptomatic: ureteritis, Bartholinitis and discharge.	Young age Other UTI Multiple partners Drug or commerical sex user/worker	Greenish-yellow discharge Inflamed Bartholin's glands Endocervical bleeding fragility (rare) Nothing common

Diagnosis	Treatment	Image
Swab Ph testing < 4.5 10% KOH prep: mycelia and spores	Prevention: loose fitting underwear, non-biologic soaps, good hygiene. Symptoms: topical antifungal such as clotrimazole. Treatment: oral or pessary antifungal such as clotrimazole.	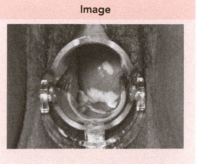
Gardnerella vaginalis on swab Ph > 4.5 Positive 'whiff test' on 10% KOH prep and clue cells (pictured) on microscopy.	None if asymptomatic. If pregnant treatment recommended. If symptomatic – metronidazole first line Rx.	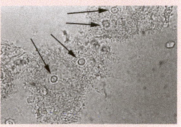
Urine nucleic acid amplification test (NAAT) is now gold standard.	Doxycycline 100 mg BD 7/7 or single dose azithromycin (often when treating gonorrhoea recommend giving concurrent chlamydia treatment)	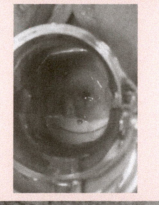
Urine nucleic acid amplification (NAAT).	Rx: simple acute infection – as above. Upper genital infection require longer courses	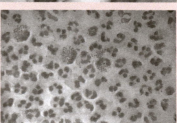
Urine NAAT now first line Swab and microscopy – gram-negative diplococci – for resistance testing and monitoring strains	Test and treat Test for other STIS Single-dose IM ceftriaxone plus azithromycin for chlamydia – before results	

Disease	Symptoms	Risk factors	Signs
Gonorrhoea (male) Neisseria gonorrhoeae	90–95% men symptomatic: symptoms appear 2–10 d after sex Dysuria, frequency, copious greenish, yellow white discharge from the penis. Can be rectal. (the clap)	As above	Copious discharge Rarely – balanitis, epidydimo-orchitis
Genital warts (condylomata acuminata)	HPV-virus – flesh-coloured, flat lesion to large cauliflower-shaped structures F: around vagina and cervix M: usually tip of penis, sometimes shaft, scrotum or anus	Sexual contact with human papilloma virus 6 and 11 (note different strain to cervical carcinoma) anoreceptive and anodigital sex	Lesions as described In HIV and immunocompromised – giant papillomas occur May be pigmented, usually multiple, may be pedunculated
Genital herpes (HSV-2 occ HSV-1)	Usually asymptomatic Flu-like prodrome 5/7, then neuropathic pain. Painful ulcers, 2/52 after sex Dysuria	HIV infection Prev STIs MSM Multiple sexual partners	Tiny painful, erythematous, vesicles on labia, vagina, cervix and thighs Often local oedema and palpable inguinal nodes
Trichomoniasis (Trichomonas vaginalis)	F: 10–50% asymptomatic M: asymptomatic usually 7–28 days post exposure Profuse frothy, greenish discharge and dysuria	Sexual transmission	Punctate 'strawberry spots' on cervix and inflamed vaginal wall

Diagnosis	Treatment	Image
As above	As above	
Clinical examination If unusual presentation biopsy is indicated to rule out malignancy	5% of warts are caused by HPV 16 and 18 – these *are* associated with cervical carcinoma	
Viral swab and PCR for typing Serology is useful in special circumstances	Symptomatic – topical anagelsia Aciclovir 400 mg TDS 5/7 – shortens severity and duration if given early onset. No cure.	
NAAT where available High vaginal swab and wet prep – visible trichmonads Swab ph > 5 Uretheral culture for men	Metronidazoe or tinadazole. Treat partners.	

Disease	Symptoms	Risk factors	Signs
Syphilis (Treponema pallidum)	Primary – painless single chancre – after 21 d from exposure – heals after 4 weeks Secondary: papulosquamous rash, non-pruritic, hands and soles – condylmata lata – may present as acute febrile flu-like illness – 'snail-track' ulcers Tertiary syphilis: > 2 years – aortic regurg, dementia, tabes dorsalis and paralysis	HIV positive MSM (recent epidemic)	See symptoms.

Features of Trichomoniasis

MNEMONIC: FIVE FS OF TRICHOMONIASIS

Flagella-shaped protozoan
Frothy discharge
intra-uterine Fishy odour (occasionally)
Fornication (a STD)
Flagyl (treated with metronidazole)

COMMUNICATION SKILLS

☐☐☐ **Safe Sex**   Educate the patient about the dangers of unprotected intercourse.

☐☐☐ **Rapport**   Establish and maintain rapport with the patient and demonstrate listening skills.

☐☐☐ **Response**   React positively to and acknowledge the patient's emotions.

☐☐☐ **Fluency**   Speak fluently and do not use jargon.

☐☐☐ **Summarise**   Check with the patient and deliver an appropriate summary.

'This is Ms Frankin, who is complaining of a 2-week history of a vulval itch, redness and discharge. She describes the discharge as thick and odourless and it is cheese-like in consistency. She does not have any associated symptoms or pain. She is currently engaged in a long-term stable relationship that has lasted for over three years and uses the pill regularly. She has never been treated for STDs nor does her partner describe any

Diagnosis	Treatment	Image
Initial screening: 1. EIA for IgM syphilis – measures exposure – not stage 2. VDRL – demonstrates stage and activity – cross-reacts with lupus 3. Dark ground microscopy to demonstrate T pallidum	IM Benzathine (penicillin) 2nd line – oral azithromycin For late/tertiary syphilis – benzathine penicillin for 3/52.	

symptoms of them. She was prescribed a course of antibiotics 1 month ago by her GP for a chest infection. She is deeply concerned that this is an STD and is worried that her partner is being unfaithful. In view of her history I suspect that this is candidiasis, however, I would like to perform an endocervical swab, HVS and urinary NAAT to rule out other differentials.'

EXAMINER'S EVALUATION

1 2 3 4 5

☐ ☐ ☐ ☐ ☐ Overall assessment of taking a sexual history
☐ ☐ ☐ ☐ ☐ Role player's score
          Total mark out of 38

2.2 SEXUAL HEALTH: HIV TEST COUNSELLING

INSTRUCTIONS

Mr D has recently returned from a trip to Thailand. He has presented to you complaining of a urethral discharge and is requesting a HIV test. Take a brief sexual history and give him the appropriate advice.

INTRODUCTION

1 2 3

☐☐☐ **Introduction** — Introduce yourself. Elicit the patient's name, age and occupation. Establish rapport.

☐☐☐ **Patient Agenda** — Establish why the patient has booked the appointment. Elicit patient's ideas, concerns and expectations.

'I am going to ask you a few personal questions to find out more about your problem. The questions may be embarrassing, but you do not have to answer them if you do not wish to. We ask these questions of all our patients and everything that you say will remain strictly confidential.'

SEXUAL HISTORY

☐☐☐ **Symptoms** — 'Do you have any discharge? Any fevers? Any urinary symptoms?'

☐☐☐ **Contacts** — 'Do you have a regular partner? Male or female? Any casual partners?'

HIV Risk-Specific Questions

Have you ever had a partner:
- with known HIV?
- from Subsaharan Africa or East Asia?
- who was a sex worker?
- who is bisexual?
- who injected drugs?

☐☐☐ **Types of SI** — 'When was the last time you had sexual intercourse (SI)? What type of intercourse did you have? Anal or vaginal?'

☐☐☐ **Contraception** — 'Did you use any form of contraception? Condoms?'

☐☐☐ **Other Activity** — 'Have you ever used intravenous drugs? Have you ever shared needles? Have you ever had a blood transfusion?'

□□□   **Past History**   'Do you suffer from any STDs? Have you ever had a HIV test before?'

□□□   **Drug History**   'Are you using any medicines? Do you have any allergies?'

HIV TESTING

□□□   **Understanding**   Elicit patient's understanding of HIV and testing.

'Have you ever had a HIV test before? Can you please tell me what you understand by HIV?'

□□□   **HIV and AIDS**   Explain in clear and simple terms the difference between HIV and AIDS.

'HIV is a virus that invades the body and weakens its defences against other infections. It can be passed in different ways, the most common being through unprotected sexual intercourse (between male and female or male and male) or by sharing infected needles. AIDS is a condition which is caused by HIV and is characterised by specific infections which infect the body as a result of the weakened immune system. The time period between HIV and developing AIDS varies from person to person and can often be many years.'

□□□   **HIV Test**   Explain how the HIV test works.

'We will take some blood from your arm and send this to the laboratory for analysis. When a person has HIV, the body produces antibodies that we can test for. If these antibodies are present, it means that HIV has been detected; if not, it means you do not have HIV.'

□□□   **Window Period**   Give appropriate advice regarding a possible negative test.

'It is important to appreciate that it can take up to 3 months after being infected with HIV for these antibodies to be produced. In essence we are assessing your HIV status 3 months ago. If you were recently infected because of unprotected sex, then the antibodies may not necessarily be present and we may get a negative result. This is known as the 'window period' and we may need to repeat the test in a few months to be sure of your status.'

□□□   **Test Results**   Explain how he will be informed of results.

'As I mentioned previously, everything that we have discussed remains confidential. The same applies for your blood results. We will not ring you or write to you with your results. Rather we will send you an appointment to attend the clinic. Some clinics have the facility to text a negative result to your mobile phone. Would this be of benefit to you?'

☐☐☐ **Implications**   Explain the possible advantages and disadvantages of having the test.

'Before taking the HIV test you may wish to consider what implications the results may have for you. One of the advantages of doing the test includes knowing whether you have HIV or not. If positive, then we can commence treatment immediately. Although treatment is not curative, most patients on medication live a normal life. Also, by knowing your status you can take precautions from spreading the virus to your partner. However, by knowing your status, this may have a negative impact on your relationship with your partner and you may also have to inform your insurance company.'

☐☐☐ **Support Group**   Enquire about support network and whether he would like more counselling.

'If the results are positive, is there anyone from your friends or family you think you can talk to? We have specially trained professionals who can counsel you if the test is positive. I can put them in touch with you if you think that may help.'

FINISHING OFF

☐☐☐ **Understanding**   Confirm patient understands what has been discussed. Encourage questions and deal with concerns accordingly.

☐☐☐ **Follow-Up**   Mention the need for an out-patient follow-up to review symptoms.

Offer Leaflet   Close the interview and offer HIV information leaflet.

EXAMINER'S EVALUATION

1 2 3 4 5

☐☐☐☐☐ Overall assessment of explaining pre-assessment HIV testing

Total mark out of 26

2.3   SEXUAL HEALTH: MALE CONDOM

INSTRUCTIONS

You are a medical student on an attachment in a family planning clinic. You have been asked to see a patient who wants advice on how to put on a condom correctly. Elicit any concerns and give the appropriate instructions using the plastic training model provided. You will be marked on your communication skills, practical skills and the information given.

INTRODUCTION

1 2 3

☐☐☐   **Introduction**   Introduce yourself. Elicit the patient's name, age and occupation. Establish rapport with him.

'I understand that you have attended the family planning clinic today to find out more about contraception? Before I discuss this topic, I would like to ask you some questions.'

☐☐☐   **Ideas**   What do you already know about using a condom?
☐☐☐   **Concerns**   Do you have any issues or concerns you would like to raise regarding using condoms?

EXPLANATION

☐☐☐   **Mechanism**   Explain in simple terms what the condom is and how it works.

'The condom is a barrier method of contraception. This means that it works by preventing the sperm from reaching the egg. It fits over the erect penis and is made out of thin latex rubber.'

☐☐☐   **Benefits**   Explain the benefits of using a condom.

'Wearing condoms greatly reduces chances of pregnancy. They also provide considerable protection against sexually transmitted infections (STIs), including HIV, but this protection is not 100%.'

☐☐☐   **Efficacy**   Explain to the patient the efficacy and failure rate.

'When used correctly, a condom is about 98% effective. This means only 2 in every 100 women would get pregnant in the course of a year. This is more effective than other forms of contraception, such as withdrawal or using spermicide on its own.'

☐☐☐ **Partner** Explain that condom use should be discussed with partner and put on before any genital contact.

'It is important that you discuss with your partner your wish to use condoms. It is important that you put the condom on before there is any genital contact between you and your partner.'

Quality Stress the importance of using British kite-marked condoms which have undergone thorough quality checks.

☐☐☐ **Expiry Date** Advise the patient to check the expiry date on the condoms and not to use them if they have expired.

Damage Advise the patient to check the condom for damage and not to inadvertently tear it with nails or rings when removing it from its packet.

Explaining use of a Condom

Advise the patient to expel the air from the teat and then demonstrate how to successfully roll on a condom on a model. Check for the kite and expiry date before using it. Be careful when opening packet not to inadvertently damage the condom.

☐☐☐ **Method** Advise the patient to expel the air from the teat and then demonstrate how to successfully roll on a condom on a model.

'It is important to squeeze the air out of the 'teat' at the end, otherwise the semen will not be able to collect or enter it if it is full of air. Now roll the condom onto the erect penis, as shown on this model. Do not try putting it on before the penis is erect. Roll it down to the base of the penis, and hold the base down as you penetrate.'

☐☐☐ **Lubricants** Recommend the patient to avoid oil-based lubricants, such as K-Y jelly or Vaseline, which can weaken the condom and predispose it to tears.

☐☐☐ **Withdrawal** State the importance of holding condom onto base of penis during withdrawal and when removing it to ensure that it has not spilt.

'As soon as you've climaxed, hold the condom firmly onto the base of your penis with your fingers, and withdraw from the vagina, taking care that no fluid is spilt. This is very important. You should check that the condom has not been damaged because this would mean that there is a possibility that semen has escaped and entered the vagina.'

Dispose		Advise the patient to remove the condom, wrap it in paper or tissue, and dispose of it in a bin. Warn the patient it is not advisable to reuse a condom. If he wishes to have sexual intercourse again he should wash his penis and use a new condom.
☐☐☐	**Fails**	Inform the patient of the availability of emergency contraception if the condom is unsuccessful.

'If the condom tears or you discover that it tore during intercourse, or it slipped or anything else happened, your partner should consult the GP or the family planning clinic as soon as possible, where emergency contraception can be provided.'

CLOSING

☐☐☐	**Understanding**	Check and confirm for patient's understanding.
☐☐☐	**Questions**	Respond appropriately to patient's questions.
	Leaflet	Offer to give them more information in the form of a handout. Advise that the leaflet contains much of the information you have mentioned.

COMMUNICATION SKILLS

☐☐☐	**Rapport**	Establish and maintain rapport and demonstrate listening skills.
☐☐☐	**Fluency**	Speak fluently and do not use jargon.
☐☐☐	**Summarise**	Check with patient and deliver an appropriate summary.

EXAMINER'S EVALUATION

1 2 3 4 5
☐☐☐☐☐ Overall assessment of explaining the use of a condom
☐☐☐☐☐ Role player's score
Total mark out of 29

2.4   SEXUAL HEALTH: COMBINED ORAL CONTRACEPTIVE PILL

INSTRUCTIONS

You are a foundation year House Officer in a general practice. Ms Johnson has asked to be started on the oral contraceptive pill. Elicit any concerns she has and give appropriate instructions. You will be marked on your communication skills and the information given.

INTRODUCTION

1 2 3

☐☐☐ **Introduction**   Introduce yourself. Elicit the patient's name, age and occupation. Establish rapport with her.

☐☐☐ **Ideas**   Why do you want to start using the oral contraceptive pill? What do you understand about the oral contraceptive pill?

☐☐☐ **Concerns**   Do you have any specific concerns regarding the oral contraceptive pill?

ASSOCIATED HISTORY

☐☐☐ **Sexual History**   Are you currently sexually active? Are you using any forms of contraception? What type have you been using and for how long? Have you been using it occasionally or all the time? Have there been any problems with the current type or method?

☐☐☐ **STIs**   Have you or your partner ever had a sexually transmitted infection, such as chlamydia, gonorrhoea or syphilis? Was it successfully treated?

☐☐☐ **Menstrual History**   When was your last period (LMP)? How long do your cycles last? Are your cycles regular? Do you have any pain or bleeding?

☐☐☐ **Obstetrics History**   Do you have any children? Are you currently breast-feeding? Is there any chance that you could be pregnant?

SUITABILITY AND CONTRAINDICATIONS

☐☐☐ **Explain**   'I need to ask you a few questions to find out if the pill is suitable for you or whether you need some other form of contraception.'

MEDICAL ADVICE

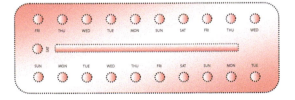

Oral Contraceptive Pill (OCP)

OCP should be taken continuously for 21 days without interruption. Then allow for a 7-day break. The pill is not suitable for all patients.

UKMEC Guidelines on Oral Contraceptive Pill Prescription (2009)

Divides patient into categories depending on risk

		Combined pill (CHC)	Progestogen-only pill
Category 1	No contraindications or restrictions	Gestational diabetes	Gestational diabetes, Obesity
Category 2	A condition where the advantages of using the method generally outweigh the theoretical or proven risks	BMI 30–35, migraine without aura	Current/history of VTE, migraine with aura, any diabetes
Category 3	A condition where the theoretical or proven risks usually outweigh the advantages of using the method. The provision of a method requires expert clinical judgement and/or referral to a specialist contraceptive provider, since use of the method is not usually recommended unless other more appropriate methods are not available or not acceptable	Smoker (< 15/day + > 35 years old), HTN, BMI > 35, risk factors for arterial disease, DM with vascular disease, cervical cancer, immobility, BRCA1 positive	Stroke, liver tumours, antiphospholipid syndrome
Category 4	A condition which represents an unacceptable health risk if the contraceptive method is used	Breast-feeding (< 6 wk postpartum), PE, DVT, IHD, CVA, migraine with aura, breast cancer, severe cirrhosis and liver tumours, smoker (> 15/day + > 35 years old), recent major surgery with immobilisation, antiphospholipid	
Drugs reducing efficacy	Rifampicin, carbamazepine, phenytoin, phenobarbitone, antibiotics, acute alcohol		

http://www.fsrh.org/pdfs/UKMEC2009.pdf

Overall – if OCP is contraindicated, POP tends to be the better option.

☐☐☐ **Mechanism** — Explain in simple terms how the contraceptive pill works.

'The combined oral contraceptive pill contains two hormones, oestrogen and progesterone, which are similar to the two the body naturally produces. It works by changing the body's hormone balance so that you do not release an egg each month from your ovary. It also makes it difficult for sperm to enter the womb to fertilise an egg and thins the uterus lining making it difficult for a fertilised egg to attach to.'

☐☐☐ **Method** — Explain to the patient how to take the combined oral contraceptive pill.

'Begin the pill on the first day of your next period. Then take the pill at the same time once a day for the next 21 days. Take a break for 7 days, during which time you may have a withdrawal bleed. However, during this break you will continue to be protected as long as you restart the next pack on time.'

☐☐☐ **Efficacy** — Explain to the patient the efficacy and failure rate.

'If taken properly, the pill is 99% successful in preventing pregnancy. However, you need to take the pill regularly and at the same time each day.'

☐☐☐ **Mishap** — Inform the patient what will happen if she misses a single pill.

'If you miss a pill, the advice we give is to carry on taking your regular pills and take the missed pill as soon as possible. You will not need to use protective barrier methods or an emergency contraceptive pill.'

'If you vomit within 3 hours of taking a pill, take another pill as soon as possible. If you are able to keep this pill down then you will continue to be protected from pregnancy.'

Guidelines for 'Missed Pill Rule'

Missed a pill (24-48 hours late)	Take the missed pill as soon as possible and continue taking the remaining pills at the regular time, even if taken at same time. No barrier contraception required.
> 48 hours late	Take the last missed pill and continue taking the remaining pills as usual. However, abstinence or condoms should be used.
If in week 1 when missed pills	The patient should consider emergency contraception if she has missed pills in the first week and had unprotected sex.
If in week 2 when missed pills	No need for emergency contraception
If in week 3 when missed pills	Start the next pack without a break – no need for emergency contraception

☐☐☐   **Advantages**   Explain to the patient the benefits of taking the pill.

'The pill is a very effective form of contraception. It often makes periods lighter, less painful and more regular. It reduces the risks of developing certain cancers such as ovarian and endometrial cancer.'

☐☐☐   **Disadvantages**   Explain to the patient the disadvantages of taking the pill.

'Most women who take the pill do not develop any side effects. However, common side effects can include nausea, headache, weight gain and mood alterations. It is also known to be associated with an increased risk of developing blood clots in the legs (DVT) and lung (PE). There is also a slightly increased risk of developing breast and cervical cancer.'

STIs

'It is also important to be aware that the pill does not protect against sexually transmitted infections and so will require barrier protection with condoms in addition if at risk.'

Side Effects of Oral Contraceptives

MNEMONIC: 'CONTRACEPTIVES'

Cholestatic jaundice
Oedema (corneal)
Nasal congestion
Thromboembolism (DVT, PE)
Raised BP
Acne, **A**lopecia, **A**naemia
CVA, TIA
Elevated blood sugar (DM)
Porphyria, **P**igmentation, **P**ancreatitis
Thyroid dysfunction
Intracranial hypertension
Vomiting (progesterone only)
Erythema nodosum, **E**xtrapyramidal effects
Sensitivity to light

Interaction   Explain to the patient the common drug interactions that reduce the efficacy of the pill (antibiotics, anti-TB drugs, antiepileptic medication).

'There are a number of drugs that can reduce the effectiveness of the pill. It is important to inform your GP or your pharmacist that you are taking the pill when you take other medications such as common antibiotics, anti-epileptic medication and treatment for tuberculosis. You may need to use additional forms of contraception (condom) for at least 2 weeks.'

☐☐☐ **Alternatives**   Suggest other forms of contraception if the patient is not suited to using the oral contraceptive pill. Explain to the patient the reasons for the incompatibility.

CLOSING

☐☐☐ **Understanding**   Check and confirm that the patient understands the instructions.
☐☐☐ **Questions**   Respond appropriately to the patient's questions.
           Leaflet   Offer to give her more information in the form of a handout. Advise that the leaflet contains much of the information you have mentioned.

COMMUNICATION SKILLS

☐☐☐ **Rapport**   Establish and maintain rapport and demonstrate listening skills.
☐☐☐ **Fluency**   Speak fluently and do not use jargon.
☐☐☐ **Summarise**   Check with the patient and deliver an appropriate summary.

EXAMINER'S EVALUATION

1 2 3 4 5
☐☐☐☐☐ Assessment of explaining the combined pill
☐☐☐☐☐ Role player's score
        Total mark out of 34

2.5   SEXUAL HEALTH: EMERGENCY CONTRACEPTIVE PILL

INSTRUCTIONS

A 15-year-old girl visits you in the A&E department. She appears frightened. She states that her previous form of contraception has failed and wants emergency contraception. Deal with her request appropriately.

NOTE

It is unlawful for doctors to provide contraceptive advice and treatment to a child under the age of 16 without parental consent unless he or she is 'Fraser competent'. The child can give consent to treatment only if she understands its nature, purpose and hazards and if the proposed treatment is in the child's best interest. Also, reasonable efforts have to be made to persuade the child to consult her parents.

HISTORY

1 2 3

□□□ **Introduction**   Introduce yourself. Elicit the patient's name, age and occupation. Establish rapport with her.

□□□ **Ideas**   'Why do you want to use the emergency contraceptive pill?'

□□□ **Concerns**   'Do you have any specific issues or concerns you would like to raise regarding the emergency contraceptive pill?'

ASSOCIATED HISTORY

□□□ **Sexual History**   Take a detailed sexual history, including the time and type of intercourse and the reason for failure.

Time   'When was the last time you had sexual intercourse? Several hours or days ago?'

Type   'Did you practise penetrative sex? Did you use protection? What type did you use (condoms, oral contraceptive pill, the diaphragm)?'

Mishap   'Was there a failure with the contraception (condom split, hole in diaphragm, forget to take pill)? Has this ever occurred in the past?'

□□□ **Menstrual Hist.**   'When was your last period (LMP)? How long do your cycles normally last? Are your cycles regular?'

Obstetrics Hist.   'Do you think you are pregnant? Have you been pregnant in the past?'

Medical History   'Do you suffer from any medical illnesses? Have you ever been admitted to hospital?'

Drug History   'Do you take any medications? Are you on any oral contraceptive pills?'

SUITABILITY AND CONTRAINDICATIONS

☐☐☐ **Explain**   Ascertain whether the patient has any contraindications for taking this form of contraception. Use the table below to guide you.

Contraindications of Emergency Contraceptive Pill (ECP)

Pregnancy, vaginal bleeding, arterial disease, liver adenoma, porphyria.

MEDICAL ADVICE

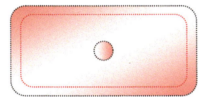

Emergency Contraception

The emergency contraceptive pill should be taken within 72 hours (Levonelle) or 120 hours (ellaOne) of unprotected sexual intercourse.

☐☐☐ **Mechanism**   Explain in simple terms how the emergency contraception works.

'The emergency contraceptive pill contains a high dose of a progestogen hormone that is similar to what the body naturally produces. It works by changing the body's hormone balance and therefore prevents or postpones an egg from being released (ovulation) and makes it more difficult for the fertilised egg to settle in the womb.'

☐☐☐ **Method**   Explain to the patient how to take the emergency contraceptive pill.

'Take the pill as soon as possible after unprotected sex. It should be taken within 72–120 hours of intercourse.'

☐☐☐ **Efficacy**   Explain to the patient the efficacy and failure rate.

'We advise all patients that the emergency contraceptive pill should be used only in an emergency as it is not as effective as other forms of contraception. It prevents around 95% of pregnancies from developing if it is taken within 24 hours of unprotected sex; and the sooner it is taken, the more effective it is.'

Efficacy of Emergency Contraception (Levonorgestrel)

Time after intercourse	% of pregnancies prevented
< 24 hours	95
24–48 hours	85
48–72 hours	58

☐☐☐ **Side Effects**   Explain to the patient the side effects of taking the emergency contraceptive pill.

'Side effects include feeling nauseous, vomiting, breast tenderness, headaches, dizziness and tiredness. Often side effects are mild and tend to disappear after a few hours. If you are sick and vomit within 3 hours of taking the pill then you will require a replacement dose.'

Period   Explain to the patient possible alteration of her monthly cycle.

'By taking this pill your next period may be a few days earlier or later than expected. However, do visit your GP or a doctor if your next period is more than 7 days later than expected, as you may require a pregnancy test.'

Abdo. Pain   Explain to the patient the warning symptoms of ectopic pregnancy.

'Visit your doctor directly if you notice any lower abdominal pains or vaginal bleeding over the next 2–6 weeks (ectopic pregnancy).'

☐☐☐ **Alternatives**   Suggest other forms of emergency contraception including the intra-uterine device.

'The IUD or intra-uterine device works by stopping an egg from being fertilised or implanted in the womb. It can be fitted up to 5 days after unprotected sex and is more effective (prevents 98% of pregnancies) than the emergency contraceptive pill. However, it is considered more invasive than the pill.'

☐☐☐ **Contraception**   Explain that the emergency contraceptive pill should not replace her usual form of contraception; rather it should be used solely for emergencies.

☐☐☐ **Education**   Stress the importance of practising safe sex with contraception.

☐☐☐ **Pregnancy Test**   Offer the patient a pregnancy test prior to prescribing the emergency contraceptive pill.

CLOSING

☐☐☐ **Understanding** Confirm that the patient has understood what you have explained to her.

☐☐☐ **Questions** Respond appropriately to the patient's questions.

Leaflet Offer to give her more information in the form of a handout. Advise that the leaflet contains much of the information you have mentioned.

COMMUNICATION SKILLS

☐☐☐ **Rapport** Establish and maintain rapport and demonstrate listening skills.

☐☐☐ **Fluency** Speak fluently and do not use jargon.

☐☐☐ **Summarise** Check with patient and deliver an appropriate summary.

EXAMINER'S EVALUATION

1 2 3 4 5

☐☐☐☐☐ Assessment of explaining emergency pill

☐☐☐☐☐ Role player's score

Total mark out of 33

2.6   SEXUAL HEALTH: INTRAMUSCULAR CONTRACEPTION

INSTRUCTIONS

You are a foundation year House Officer in a general practice. Mrs Shakespeare is a 30-year-old teacher who is interested in taking Depo-Provera and would like to know more about it. Deal with her request appropriately.

HISTORY

1 2 3

☐☐☐ **Introduction**   Introduce yourself. Elicit the patient's name, age and occupation. Establish rapport with her.

☐☐☐ **Ideas**   Why do you want to use Depo-Provera?

☐☐☐ **Concerns**   Do you have any specific issues or concerns you would like to raise regarding this form of contraception?

Depo-Provera (Injectable Contraception)

Depo-Provera is a progestogen-containing contraceptive injection. The active ingredient is 150 mg of depot medroxyprogesterone acetate (DMPA). It is given every 3 months (12–13 weeks) intramuscularly. It works by inhibiting follicular development and preventing ovulation. Under 'perfect attendance' the first year failure rate is 0.3%. However, its average efficacy is 97%. Because of its prolonged action it should never be given without counselling the patient

---

SUITABILITY AND CONTRAINDICATIONS

☐☐☐ **Explain**   Ascertain whether the patient has any contraindications for taking this form of contraception. Use the information below to guide you.

Contraindications of Depo-Provera (see UKMEC guidelines for full detail)

Absolute	Pregnancy (delay 6 weeks postpartum before commencing), DVT, PE, CVA, serious liver disease (hepatitis, cirrhosis, tumours), breast cancer, undiagnosed vaginal bleeding, known hypersensitivity to Depo-Provera

MEDICAL ADVICE

☐☐☐ **Mechanism**   Explain in simple terms how Depo-Provera works.

'Depo-Provera is a form of contraception that is delivered as an injection. It contains progesterone (medroxyprogesterone acetate), which is a chemical that is naturally found in your body. It works in three different ways. Firstly, it puts your ovaries to sleep, preventing the release of an egg. Secondly, it thins the lining of your womb, preventing the egg from attaching securely. Finally, it makes the mucus in the neck of your womb thicker, preventing sperm from reaching your womb.'

☐☐☐ **Efficacy**   Explain to the patient the efficacy and failure rate.

'It is very effective and has a failure rate of less than 1%, which means that in every 100 sexually active women using it, only 1 on average will become pregnant over the course of a year.'

☐☐☐ **Method**   Explain to the patient how the Depo-Provera is administered.

'The injection is given into the buttock every 12 weeks. If it is given in the first 5 days of your menstrual cycle it provides immediate protection. On any other day you will require extra protection for 7 days using barrier methods, such as the condom.'

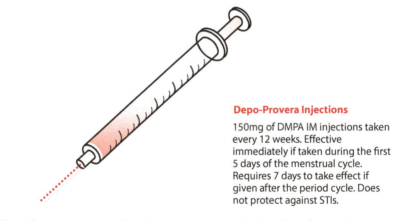

Depo-Provera Injections

150mg of DMPA IM injections taken every 12 weeks. Effective immediately if taken during the first 5 days of the menstrual cycle. Requires 7 days to take effect if given after the period cycle. Does not protect against STIs.

☐☐☐ **Advantages**   Explain to the patient the benefits of using intramuscular contraception.

'Depo-Provera provides long-lasting protection against pregnancy without the side effects of the combined pill. It is also highly effective and does not interfere with sex. It is safe while breast-feeding and offers some protection against cancer of the womb.'

☐☐☐ **Disadvantages**   Explain to the patient the disadvantages of using intramuscular contraception.

'It is important to note that 9 out of 10 women who take Depo-Provera will stop having periods after a year of use, whilst others may experience irregular periods. Once the injections have stopped, there is usually a delay of up to 18 months before fertility returns fully.'

Side Effects

'Side effects include headaches, weight gain, breast tenderness and mood swings.'

STIs

'Depo-Provera does not protect against STIs, so you will require barrier protection with condoms in addition if you are at risk.'

CLOSING

☐☐☐ **Alternatives**   Suggest other forms of contraception if the patient is not suited to use Depo-Provera or the treatment is contraindicated. Explain to the patient the reasons for such incompatibility.

☐☐☐ **Understanding**   Confirm that the patient has understood what you have explained to her.

☐☐☐ **Questions**   Respond appropriately to the patient's questions.

Leaflet   Offer to give her more information in the form of a handout. Advise that the leaflet contains much of the information you have mentioned.

COMMUNICATION SKILLS

☐☐☐ **Rapport**   Establish and maintain rapport and demonstrate listening skills.

☐☐☐ **Fluency**   Speak fluently and do not use jargon.

☐☐☐ **Summarise**   Check with the patient and deliver an appropriate summary.

EXAMINER'S EVALUATION

1 2 3 4 5

☐☐☐☐☐ Assessment of explaining the Depo-Provera method

☐☐☐☐☐ Role player's score

Total mark out of 28

2.7   SEXUAL HEALTH: CONTRACEPTIVE IMPLANT

INSTRUCTIONS

You are a foundation year House Officer in general practice. Mrs Butt is a 30-year-old PR executive who is interested in using the Implanon device and would like to know more about it. Deal with her request appropriately.

HISTORY

1 2 3

☐☐☐ **Introduction**   Introduce yourself. Elicit the patient's name, age and occupation. Establish rapport.

☐☐☐ **Ideas**   Why do you want to use the Implanon device?

☐☐☐ **Concerns**   Do you have any specific issues or concerns you would like to raise regarding this form of contraception?

Implanon (Contraceptive Implant)

Implanon is a single-rod contraceptive subdermal implant that is inserted into the medial aspect of the non-dominant upper arm. It releases approximately 40 mcg of etonorgestrel a day over a 3-year period. It works primarily by preventing ovulation but also increases cervical mucus viscosity, inhibiting sperm penetration. The typical failure rate is 0.05% and it must be inserted by a trained health professional. Its effects are rapidly reversible, with normal fertility returning within days of its removal.

SUITABILITY AND CONTRAINDICATIONS

☐☐☐ **Explain**   Ascertain whether the patient has any contraindications for taking this form of contraception. Use the table below to guide you.

Contraindications of Implanon

Absolute	Pregnancy (delay 6 weeks postpartum before commencing), DVT, PE, CVA, serious liver disease (hepatitis, cirrhosis, tumours), breast cancer, breast-feeding (< 6 wks postpartum), undiagnosed vaginal bleeding, known hypersensitivity to Implanon

MEDICAL ADVICE

☐☐☐ **Mechanism**   Explain in simple terms how the Implanon device works.

'Implanon is a small flexible tube that is 40 mm long and 2 mm wide (the size of a matchstick) which is placed under the skin of the upper arm. It contains a chemical that is similar to the naturally occurring female sex hormone, progesterone. Progesterone is released slowly into the blood stream at a steady rate. It works by changing the body's hormone balance and therefore prevents an egg from being released (ovulation) and makes it difficult for the fertilised egg to settle in the womb by making the lining of the womb thinner. It also makes the mucus in the neck of the womb thicker, preventing the sperm from entering the womb.'

☐ ☐ ☐   **Efficacy**   Explain to the patient the efficacy and failure rate.

'It is very effective and has a failure rate of less than 1%, which means that in 100 sexually active women using it, only 1 will become pregnant over the course of a year.'

☐ ☐ ☐   **Inserted**   Explain to the patient how the Implanon is placed.

'Implanon is put in the inner side of the upper arm. A local anaesthetic is injected to numb the skin. Then an incision is made where the implant will be placed using an applicator. The procedure can take less than a minute. Some patients may have pain and bruising for a few days.'

☐ ☐ ☐   **Protection**   Give appropriate advice regarding the insertion of the Implanon device in relation to the patient's cycle.

'If inserted in the first 5 days of your menstrual cycle it provides immediate protection. However, on any other day of your cycle, you will require extra protection for 7 days by using barrier methods, such as condoms.'

☐ ☐ ☐   **Remove**   Explain to the patient when and how the Implanon device should be removed.

'Implanon provides contraception for 3 years and requires replacing after this. In order to remove the Implanon device a small cut is made under local anaesthetic and then it is removed with small forceps.'

☐ ☐ ☐   **Advantages**   Explain to the patient the benefits of the Implanon device.

'One of the advantages of the Implanon device is that it lasts for 3 years and you do not need to worry about contraception during this time. It is extremely reliable, does not interfere with sex and is safe while you are breast-feeding. It is also rapidly reversible in that, within a very short time after its removal, your blood hormone levels return back to normal.'

☐☐☐ **Disadvantages**   Explain to the patient the disadvantages of the Implanon device.

'Some of the disadvantages include unpredictable changes to your periods. Most women experience irregular bleeding in the first year. However, after 1 year most settle back to a regular pattern. Some women experience infrequent and light periods and occasionally no periods at all (amenorrhoea).'

Side Effects

'Side effects include headaches, weight gain, breast tenderness and mood swings.'

STIs

'Implanon does not protect against STI so you will require barrier protection with condoms in addition if you are at risk of STDs.'

☐☐☐ **Alternatives**   Suggest another form of contraception if the patient is not suited to Implanon or there are contraindications for using it. Explain to the patient the reasons for her incompatibility.

CLOSING

☐☐☐ **Understanding**   Confirm that the patient has understood what you have explained to her.
☐☐☐ **Questions**   Respond appropriately to the patient's questions.
      Leaflet   Offer to give her more information in the form of a handout. Advise that the leaflet contains much of the information you have mentioned.

COMMUNICATION SKILLS

☐☐☐ **Rapport**   Establish and maintain rapport and demonstrate listening skills.
☐☐☐ **Fluency**   Speak fluently and do not use jargon.
☐☐☐ **Summarise**   Check with the patient and deliver an appropriate summary.

EXAMINER'S EVALUATION

1 2 3 4 5
☐☐☐☐☐ Assessment of explaining the Implanon device
☐☐☐☐☐ Role player's score
        Total mark out of 30

2.8   SEXUAL HEALTH: INTRA-UTERINE DEVICE (IUD)

INSTRUCTIONS

You are a foundation year House Officer in General Practice. Mrs Anderson is a 35-year-old pilot who is interested in using the intra-uterine device and would like to know more about it. Deal with her request appropriately.

INTRODUCTION

1 2 3

☐☐☐   **Introduction**   Introduce yourself. Elicit the patient's name, age and occupation. Establish rapport.

☐☐☐   **Ideas**   What do you already know about the intra-uterine device?

☐☐☐   **Concerns**   Do you have any specific issues or concerns you would like to raise regarding this form of contraception?

ASSOCIATED HISTORY

☐☐☐   **Menstrual Hist**   'When was your last period (LMP)? How long do your cycles last? Are your cycles regular? Do you have any pain or bleeding?'

☐☐☐   **STIs**   'Have you or your partner ever had a sexually transmitted infection, such as chlamydia, gonorrhoea or syphilis? Was it successfully treated?'

   Obstetric History   'Do you have any children? Are you currently breast-feeding? Is there any chance that you could be pregnant?'

SUITABILITY AND CONTRAINDICATIONS

☐☐☐   **Explain**   Ascertain whether the patient has any contraindications for using this form of contraception. Use the table below to guide you.

Contraindications of IUD

Absolute	Pregnancy, fibroids, severe anaemia, STI, unexplained vaginal bleeding, uterine malignancy, PID, copper allergy, Wilson's disease

MEDICAL ADVICE

☐☐☐   **Mechanism**   Explain in simple terms how the intra-uterine device works.

'The intra-uterine device is a small T-shaped apparatus, often containing copper, that is inserted into the womb. It is approximately the size of a matchstick, with threads that should hang out a little from your vagina. These help you to identify whether the device is in place. It works by making it difficult for the fertilised egg to settle in the womb and grow.'

☐☐☐ **Efficacy**   Explain to the patient the efficacy and failure rate.

'It is a highly effective form of contraception and tends to have a failure rate between 0.2% and 2%. This means that in 100 sexually active women using it, fewer than 2 will become pregnant over the course of a year.'

☐☐☐ **Method**   Explain to the patient how the IUD will be placed.

'The intra-uterine device can be inserted only by a trained health professional. This usually takes place during your period. While you are lying on a couch a speculum is inserted into the vagina, similar to having a smear taken. The device is then inserted through the neck of your womb. The procedure is quite straightforward but you may suffer from some slight discomfort.'

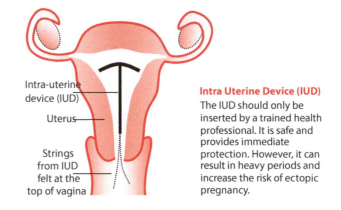

Intra-uterine
device (IUD)

Uterus

Strings
from IUD
felt at the
top of vagina

Intra Uterine Device (IUD)
The IUD should only be inserted by a trained health professional. It is safe and provides immediate protection. However, it can result in heavy periods and increase the risk of ectopic pregnancy.

☐☐☐ **Advantages**   Explain to the patient the benefits of using the intra-uterine device.

'One of the advantages of the IUD is that it is very safe. It provides immediate protection and doesn't interfere with intercourse. It also has a long lifespan of up to 8 years and can be removed at any time.'

☐☐☐ **Disadvantages** Explain to the patient the disadvantages of using the intra-uterine device.

'Some of the disadvantages include experiencing painful, heavy periods and an increased risk of developing infection or inflammation of the pelvis (PID). There is a very small possibility (1 in 1000) of the device puncturing the womb. There is also a slight chance that the device could fail and that a pregnancy takes place outside your womb (ectopic pregnancy). In this unlikely event, you should seek urgent medical advice.'

STIs

'An IUD does not protect against STIs, so you will require barrier protection with condoms in addition if you are at risk of STDs.'

Side Effects of Intra-Uterine Devices (IUDs)

MNEMONIC: 'PAIN'

Period that is late
Abdominal cramps
Increase in body temperature
Noticeable vaginal discharge

☐☐☐   **Check Threads**   Stress the importance of checking the threads of the IUD.
          Alternatives   Suggest other forms of contraception if the patient is not suited
                         to an IUD or there are contraindications for using it. Explain to
                         the patient the reasons for the incompatibility.

Contraindications for Intra-Uterine Devices

MNEMONIC: 'PLEASE DON'T EVER PUT-UP CONTRACEPTIVES':

Pregnancy, **D**UB, **E**ctopic pregnancy, **P**ID, **C**arcinoma (cervical)

CLOSING

☐☐☐   **Understanding**   Confirm that the patient has understood what you have
                         explained to her.
☐☐☐   **Questions**   Respond appropriately to her questions.
          Leaflet   Offer to give her more information in the form of a handout.
                         Advise that the leaflet contains much of the information you
                         have mentioned.

COMMUNICATION SKILLS

☐☐☐   **Rapport**   Establish and maintain rapport with her and demonstrate
                         listening skills.
☐☐☐   **Fluency**   Speak fluently and do not use jargon.
☐☐☐   **Summarise**   Check with patient and deliver an appropriate summary.

EXAMINER'S EVALUATION

1 2 3 4 5
☐☐☐☐☐   Assessment of explaining the IUD
☐☐☐☐☐   Role player's score
                Total mark out of 30

Paediatrics

3

3.1   PAEDIATRICS: PAEDIATRIC HISTORY

INSTRUCTIONS

You are a foundation year House Officer in paediatric outpatients. Mrs Cooper has brought in her 7-year-old son for an appointment. Take an appropriate history. You will be marked on your interviewing skills and ability to elicit the history.

NOTE

When taking a paediatric history, it is important to adapt your history-taking around the child's age. Certain questions become more significant for a toddler than a teenager. Ensure you address questions to both the parent and the child when appropriate.

INTRODUCTION

1 2 3

☐☐☐	**Introduction**	Introduce yourself and establish rapport.
☐☐☐	**Name and Age**	Elicit the child's name (preferred as well as official) and confirm the relationship of the adult accompanying the child. Elicit the age of the child in years and months or days and weeks for babies.

HISTORY

☐☐☐	**Complaint**	Elicit all the patient's presenting complaints.
☐☐☐	**History**	'When did it first start? What did you first notice? When was the child last well? Did it come on suddenly or gradually? Is it getting better or worse? Have you ever had it before? Has the child been exposed to unwell individuals (e.g. siblings)?'
	Cough	'Has he had a cough? Is it worse during the day or the night? Is it made worse by exercise? What does it sound like (barking, a whoop, wet or dry)? Is there an associated wheeze? Any sputum or phlegm?'
	Fever	'Have you been feeling hot? How high did the temperature go? Is it a swinging fever? Any shaking (rigors) or fits (seizures)? Have you taken any medication? Any headaches or intolerance to light (photophobia)? Any rashes (face/trunk/nappy area)? What does the rash look like? Does it change colour when pressed (blanching/non-blanching)?'

Number of Days into Illness Rash Appears

MNEMONIC: 'VERY SICK PEOPLE MUST TAKE EARLY RETIREMENT'

Day 1 **V**aricella (10–21d incubation)
Day 2 **S**carlet fever (1–7d incubation)
Day 3 **P**ox (small) (12d incubation)
Day 4 **M**easles (7 to 21d incubation)
Day 5 **T**yphus (epidemic) (7–14d incubation period)
Day 6 **E**nteric fever (typhoid) (3–30d)
Day 7 **R**ubella (incubation period 14–23d)

	D and V	'How many times has he passed stools (neonates – wet nappies)? Are the stools loose, watery or fully formed? Any blood, mucus or tummy pain? Is there any pain associated with feeding? Does he pass urine everyday? How many times has he vomited? Is the vomiting related to meals? Is there projectile vomiting (pyloric stenosis)? Is there any associated fever? Does he feel nauseous? What colour is the vomit? Is there any blood?'
	Seizures	'Did he have a fever before the fit? How long did it last for? Did he bite his tongue? Did he wet himself or lose consciousness? Were his limbs jerking? Did he feel sleepy or drowsy afterwards?'
	Systemic Review	'Does he have any pain anywhere? Has he been constipated? Is he playing normally? Has he passed urine? Has he been drowsy or irritable? Does he have any lumps anywhere? Any sweats?'
☐☐☐	**Concerns**	'Do you have any particular concerns or worries about the symptoms your child is experiencing? Do you know what may be causing them?'
☐☐☐	**Impact on Life**	'How have these symptoms affected his life? And his family?'

Principles of Good Paediatric History Taking

1. Listen attentively to the parents: Elicit their ideas and worries regarding their child's illness.
2. Take a thorough history: Ascertain the chronological order of the symptoms and explore each one individually, taking note of the speed of onset, duration, character and frequency of pattern. Include a detailed past medical, family, social, developmental, immunisation and birth history.
3. Engage the child: Listen to the child carefully. He/she may be able to give a surprisingly detailed account of the illness. Ensure their account of events is corroborated by their parents.
4. Tailor the history: Take into account the child's age. Use appropriate vocabulary and props (toys and teddy bears). Do not be patronising or dismiss anything the child may say.

ASSOCIATED HISTORY

☐☐☐ **Medical History**   Ascertain a history of any serious medical illnesses (asthma, epilepsy, diabetes) or operations. Any skin problems (eczema)? Has he/she ever been jaundiced or suffered from seizures? Is there a history of repeated GP or A&E attendance? Any previous SCBU admissions?

☐☐☐ **Birth History**   How was the childbirth? Were there any maternal illnesses during pregnancy (diabetes, raised blood pressure, IUGR, viral infections)? Any problems or complications (prolonged labour)? Normal or assisted delivery? Full term or early birth? Any illnesses or problems after birth (growth, heart, breathing, jaundice)?

☐☐☐ **Maternal History**   Any problems during pregnancy (oligohydramnios, pre-eclampsia, diabetes, medication, harmful substances, viral illness such as hepatitis B, varicella, HIV)? Any problems after pregnancy (over/underweight)?

Feeding   Ask when solids were introduced, whether the child was breast-fed or bottle-fed and if there were any problems during weaning. If the patient is an infant, ask the parent if the infant is being breast-fed or bottle-fed, how often they are fed and how many bottles per day.

Development   Ask for the child's red book, if appropriate. Check the child's height, weight and head circumference and record the centiles. Ask the parents if they have any concerns regarding the child's growth, weight and development. If appropriate for the child's age, ask about developmental milestones achieved so far (see Chapter 3.4 on child development).

☐☐☐ **Well-being**   What is the child's mood or demeanour usually like? Have there been any changes recently? Is the child eating and drinking normally? Does the child have any sleeping problems?

☐☐☐ **Immunisations**   Confirm with the parents which immunisations the child has had to date. Ask the parents if they have brought with them a record of immunisations.

Pedigree Symbols

○ □ Unaffected female, male	○—□ Mating: mate & female
● ■ Affected female, male	○=□ Consanguineous mating
◑ ◨ Heterozygote (carrier) of autosomal recessive disease	○—□ Mating with two female offspring
⊙ Female heterozygote in X-linked inheritance	
⊘ Deceased	○—□ Abortion
③ 3 unaffected females	

Failure to Thrive in Children

Assessing for Failure to Thrive in Young Children

The term, 'failure to thrive' is used to describe infants or toddlers whose rate of weight gain or growth is suboptimal. It is important that regular and accurate measurements of height and weight are taken and recorded over time. The values are then plotted on a centile chart, which can reveal signs of failure to thrive. A single observation out of context provides little information, but a consistent fall across two major centile lines over time is suggestive of failure to thrive.

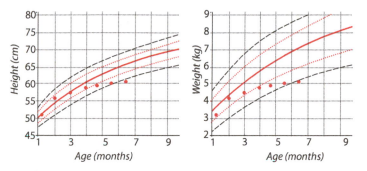

Causes of Failure to Thrive

Non-organic (80%)	Poor feeding technique, insufficient milk, economic deprivation, emotional deprivation, child neglect or abuse
Organic (20%)	
Poor calorie input	Insufficient milk, malnutrition, mechanical problems (cleft palate, CP)
Vomiting	Gastro-oesophageal reflux, pyloric stenosis, hiatus hernia, infection
Inadequate absorption	Coeliac disease, lactose intolerance, pancreatic disease (CF), IBD, giardiasis
Chronic disease	CF, CHD, CRF, renal tubular acidosis
Metabolic or endocrine	Thyroid disease, DM, GH deficiency, errors of metabolism
Syndromes	Turner's, Down's, foetal alcohol syndrome

☐☐☐ **Family History**   Are there any illnesses that run in the family (cystic fibrosis)? Are the parents related (consanguinity)? How are the other siblings? Draw a pedigree chart to assist you.

☐☐☐ **Drug History**   Does the child take any regular medication? Does he have any allergies (to medications, food, pets)?

☐☐☐ **Social History**   Take a detailed history of the home and school circumstances.
　　　　Home   Who lives at home with the child? Are there any problems at home? What do the parents do for a living? Does anyone at home smoke?

　　　　School   How are things going at school? Is the child in the appropriate year? Is he performing well? Any concerns of bullying?

COMMUNICATION SKILLS

☐☐☐ **Rapport**   Establish and maintain rapport with the child and parent whilst demonstrating listening skills.

☐☐☐ **Summarise**   Check with the patient (and parent) and deliver an appropriate summary.

'This is Johnny, a 7-year-old boy brought in by his mother, with a 3-day history of wheezing. The wheeze is worse at night and is associated with temperature and dry cough. There is no shortness of breath on exertion or whilst playing. He is eating and drinking well and passing a good volume of urine. The mother has not noticed any rash nor has the child been drowsy at any time. He suffered from eczema when he was younger, and his eldest sister suffers from asthma. He has been feeling tired and has not attended school for the last 2 days. Mum has not given any medication and is concerned that her son may be asthmatic. In view of the history, I suspect that Johnny is suffering with an upper respiratory tract infection (viral wheeze). However, I would like to exclude asthma as a possible cause.'

EXAMINER'S EVALUATION

1 2 3 4 5

☐☐☐☐☐ Overall assessment of paediatric history

☐☐☐☐☐ Role player's score

Total mark out of 28

COMMON CHILDHOOD PRESENTATIONS

Headache

Diagnosis	Symptoms	Management
Meninigitis	Fever, nausea and vomiting, decreased GCS and seizures Infants: high pitched cry, bulging fontanelle Older children: Photophobia and neck stiffness	Immediate senior review Antibiotics as soon as strong suspicion Early steroids, depending on local protocol
Tension headache	Generalised ache or tightness – mild to moderate Typically hours – can be episodic over weeks No aura or associated features	Manage underlying cause – look for poor sleep stressors at home or school
Migraine	5% of children. Throbbing, unilateral headache, temporal or frontal – moderate to severe – 1–72 hours' duration. Associated with nausea, vomiting, photophobia and visual aura (scintillating scotoma). Often positive family history. Relieved by sleep. (See below for classification.)*	Avoid triggers – bright lights, foods Analgesia and triptans for acute attacks Preventative meds – e.g. propranolol Be wary for any change in headache and treat as any of the above
Space-occupying lesion headache	Worst in morning and on lying flat Progressive and continuous over weeks to months May be associated neurology – weakness, visual changes, seizures Check for papilloedema – blurred disc margin	Urgent brain imaging Specialist assessment Seizures need to be seen by A&E
Sinusitis	Infection or inflammation of one or more paranasal sinuses (frontal, ethmoid, maxillary, sphenoid). It can be acute (< 4 weeks), subacute (4–12 weeks) or chronic (> 12 wks). Facial pain over the affected sinuses, fever, facial swelling, congestion and discharge.	Often resolves spontaenously Decongestants, anti-inflammatories and occasionally corticosteroid nasal spray or antibiotics are useful.

*Migraine Classification	
Without aura	Common migraine (5 or more episodes, headache < 72 hours, pulsating, moderate to severe, bilateral or unilateral, aggravated by movement, nausea and vomiting, photophobia and phonophobia)
With aura	Migraines that are preceded (by 30 min) with visual sensations (flashes, lines, hemianopia, blurred vision, blindness, visual hallucinations) or motor (hemiplegia) symptoms. Overall 5% of children have auras without a headache
Periodic syndrome	Childhood periodic syndromes include cyclical vomiting, abdominal migraine, benign paroxysmal vertigo of childhood – difficult to diagnose
Retinal migraine	Migraine headaches with repeated attacks of monocular visual symptoms, including scintillations, scotomata or blindness

Fits (Seizures)

Diagnosis	Symptoms	Management
Neonatal seizures	Usually focal, usually involving one limb or side of the body. Tonic-clonic generalised seizures are rare. Secondary to birth injury, infections, developmental problems or metabolic disease. Usually occur in the first few weeks post birth.	Immediate assessment in an emergency setting. Assess baby in ABC approach – consider anaesthetics if airway compromised or patient in status.
Febrile convulsions	Most common – seen in pre-school children. Associated with rapid elevations in body temperature usually associated with simple viral illness. Up to 5 years, < 15 minutes. Generalised tonic-clonic activity	Antipyretics Cooling Seeking help early if seizures persist or other neurology.
Idiopathic epilepsy	Not associated with fever – no underlying cause (e.g. no space occupying mass) Generalised – tonic-clonic, absence, myoclonic seizures Partial-simple (single limb) or complex (higher function involvement)	EEG – 50% abnormal MRI imaging Advice to avoid swimming and bathing. Not locking rooms if alone. Prophylactic anticonvulsant therapy – depending on seizure type, age, and probability of recurrence
Non-epileptiform attack disorder	Usually 'shaking' of all four limbs, associated with back arching, eyes shut tight No loss of continence, no tongue biting, no postictal state, no tonic stage	Often associated with underlying psychiatric disorder – assessment by neurologist – EEG and referral as required.

Respiratory Complaints

Diagnosis	Symptoms	Management
Upper respiratory tract infections	Common – usually viral. Exam the ears, nose and throat for evidence of bacterial infection. Always examine for quincy. Can have complications: febrile seizures.	Watchful waiting Periodic antipyretics
Asthma	Diurnal variation in symptoms, dry cough, wheeze (not always present) – exposure to irritants (dust, smoke) may reflect in pattern of symptoms – e.g better on the weekend. Commonly associated with eczema, allergies and positive family history.	Avoid smoking at home – including changing clothes (significant risk with smoke particles in clothing) Routine treatment bronchodilators May require preventative inhalers (see NICE guidance)
Common causes of cough	Asthma, postnasal drip, chronic rhinorrhoea and home irritants. If productive of sputum consider bronchiectasis: in children most likely cause is cystic fibrosis, Kartagener's or immunodeficiency	Treat the underlying cause

Rash

Diagnosis	Symptoms	Management	Image
Napkin dermatitis (nappy rash)	Occurs with irritation from wet nappies, prolonged contact with urine or faeces, infections (bacterial and candida) and other skin disorders (e.g. psoriasis).	Changing wet nappies quickly Perineal washing and drying Barrier creams	
Cradle cap	Thick, crusty, brownish rash on scalp of infants – non-itchy usually. It can spread to become seborrheic dermatitis – generalised inflammation that is self-limiting.	Oils and shampoos	
Impetigo	Highly contagious – blister > ulcerates and pus which dries to a golden brown crust. Usually itchy and spreads easily. Staphyloccous aureus commonest cause – S. pyogenes secondary.	Keep home – use separate towels Wash with water and antiseptic Occasionally requires oral/topical abx	
Atopic eczema	Red, flaky and itchy skin – following exposure to foods, allergens and irritants. Increasingly common in 15–20% school chidlren. Associated with atopy, asthma and hayfever. 50% will resolve < 2 and 50% will continue suffering.	Avoid all soaps and scented body wash Emollient and ointments 2nd line: topical steroid, antihistamine, antibacterial creams. Oral abx are reserved for systemic infections. Reduce cotton undercloths. Mittens to stop scratching	
Psoriasis	Occasionally affects joints as well – red circumscribed patches with silvery plaques. Non-itchy – typically extensor, as well as scalp. Strong familiy history – usually > 10 years old and stress factors	Treatment involves topical steroids, topical car, vitamin D preparations, phototherapy and even oral agents in extremis under specialist guidance.	

Gastrointestinal Complaints

Diagnosis	Symptoms	Management
Non-organic abdominal pain	Central, positive family history, vomiting, a tense personality and often high-achieving status. Absence: no signs, no abnormal growth and normal blood tests. Can become chronic in some cases.	Reassurance and referral to psych if needed
Appendicitis	Central abdominal pain – radiates to right iliac fossa and is worsening on moving and coughing. Beware the pain that gets better on its own – this can be a sign of perforation. Remember urine dipstick is often positive due to urethral irritation.	Urgent surgical review. May require imaging in the first instance if unclear history
Mesenteric adenitis	Typically right iliac fossa pain, sometimes history of non-specific illness preceding.	Observation and rehydration
Pyelonephritis	Loin pain and renal angle tenderness, can present very unwell – urine dipstick positive.	Targetted antibiotics – usually initially intravenous if unwell
Intussusception	Bowel prolapse into an adjacent section – common at the terminal ileum or ileo-caecal junction. < 2 years, paraoxysmal pain, vomiting, red currant jelly stool and indrawing of legs.	Urgent barium enema can help – surgery opinion plus operation is indicated

Bedwetting (Enuresis)

Enuresis is generally regarded as inappropriate voiding of urine when the child is of an age where control is expected. A more specific definition is repeated urination into bed or clothes in a child aged 5 or more years, which has occurred for a duration of 3 or more months at a frequency of at least two times a week. It usually occurs at night (nocturnal enuresis). Nocturnal enuresis occurs more commonly in boys and in lower social classes and is associated with a positive family history. Causes include a general developmental delay and stressful events (especially around the time when micturitional control is being learnt). Underlying illness or side effects of medication need to be reliably excluded before a diagnosis is made. Most children with enuresis do not suffer from psychological disorders or other illnesses, and conditions associated with urinary symptoms (e.g. urinary tract infection, diabetes) rarely present with enuresis. Treatment strategies begin with encouragement (e.g. enuresis diary, with rewards for dry nights), followed by conditioning therapy (enuresis alarm systems which detect bed wetting, sound the alarm, and cause the child to waken and go to the toilet). Drugs are used to a limited extent in the treatment of nocturnal enuresis as the rate of relapse following withdrawal of medication is high. Drugs used include tricyclic antidepressants and antidiuretics. Daytime enuresis occurs more commonly in girls and is usually due to urge incontinence secondary to bladder instability. Management involves eradicating any associated urinary infection, encouraging the child to go to the toilet more frequently and timed voiding.

3.2   PAEDIATRICS: HEADACHE HISTORY

INSTRUCTIONS

You are a foundation year House Officer in paediatrics. Mrs Ridley has brought James, an 11-year-old boy, to see you. She is very concerned about his headaches and is demanding a CT scan. Take an appropriate history and offer advice. You will be marked on your interviewing skills, ability to elicit the history and on the advice that you give.

INTRODUCTION

1 2 3

☐☐☐ **Introduction**   Introduce yourself and establish rapport.

☐☐☐ **Name and Age**   Elicit child's name and age as well as relationship to the adult.

☐☐☐ **Ideas**   Elicit patient's (mother's) ideas about what may be causing the headaches.

☐☐☐ **Concerns**   Establish any concerns (CT scan to exclude brain tumour) or fears the mother may have regarding the symptom.

FOCUSED HISTORY

☐☐☐ **Headaches**   Ask the patient (and mother) all relevant questions regarding the headaches including site, onset, character, radiation, etc. (**mnemonic – SOCRATES**).

☐☐☐ *Site*   'Where exactly is the pain? Could you please point to it? Does it affect one side or both sides of your head?'

☐☐☐ *Severity*   'How bad are these headaches? Are they affecting your schoolwork? Have you missed any days off school?'

Onset   'When did you first notice the pain? What were you doing at the time? Did it come on quickly or slowly?'

☐☐☐ *Character*   'Can you describe what the pain feels like? Does it feel like it is beating (pulsating), a needle prick (sharp) or aching (dull) pain? Does it feel like a tightening rope passing across your forehead (band-like)?'

Signs and Symptoms of Migraines

MNEMONIC: 'POUNDING'

Pulsating
HOurs (between 1 and 72 hrs)
Unilateral
Nausea
Disabling

	Radiation	'Does the pain move anywhere?'
	Relieving	'Does anything make the pain better (posture)? Does sleeping make it go away? Are the headaches better on weekends or days off school (stress/school-related)?'
☐☐☐	*Aggravating*	'Does anything make the headache worse? Such as coughing, moving your head, foods (caffeine, cheese, chocolates), flashing lights, lack of sleep?'

Triggers for Migraines

Triggers can be behavioural, environmental, dietary, chemical or hormonal	
Behavioural	Stress (school, bullying), anxiety, too much or too little sleep, missing meals
Environmental	Smoking (passive/active), bright lights, flickering lights (computer screens), loud noises, perfumes, motion sickness
Dietary	Tyramine-containing products (aged cheese, red wine, smoked fish), nitrates and nitrites (preserved meat, bacon, hotdogs, pork) and monosodium glutamate (MSG – flavour enhancer). Others include chocolate, citrus fruits, dairy products, lack of water, alcohol, caffeine (coffee, tea, colas)
Hormonal	Oral contraceptives, menstruation
Chemical	Excessive use of analgesics (NSAIDs)

	Timing	'When do the headaches come on (morning, afternoon, after school)? Do they wake you up? How long do they last for?'
	Exertion	'Is the pain worse on playing or doing sports?'
☐☐☐	*Symptoms*	'Have you noticed anything else such as feeling sick, vomiting or tummy pain? Have you had a fever or skin rash? Do get pain when you look at a strong light (photophobia) or hear loud sounds (phonophobia)? Have you had any blurred vision or flashing lights? Do you have any stiffness in your neck (meningeal irritation)? How is your concentration? Have you had any change in your behaviour (angry and irritable, sad and depressed)? Have you had any pins or needles over your face or body? Do you feel sleepy all the time (drowsiness)?'

Early Signs of Meningitis

1. pale dusky skin with cyanotic discolouration of lips
2. temperature and cold peripheries
3. severe leg pain.

☐☐☐	**Head Injury**	'Have you hit your head or had a fall recently?'
☐☐☐	**Medical History**	Ascertain a history of any past serious medical illnesses (asthma, epilepsy, diabetes) or operations. Has he ever been jaundiced or suffered from seizures? Is there any history of repeated GP or A&E attendances? Does the patient wear glasses

(or have difficulty reading the blackboard)? When was the last eye test?

☐☐☐ **Family History**   Does anyone in the family suffer with migraines? Are there any inherited family disorders?

Drug History   Current medications and what medicines have been attempted for the headache. Any drug allergies?

☐☐☐ **Social History**   Any stress at home or bullying at school? Is the child in the appropriate year? Is he performing well or have there been concerns with poor performance?

COMMUNICATION SKILLS

☐☐☐ **Rapport**   Establish and maintain rapport with the child and parent whilst demonstrating listening skills.

☐☐☐ **Response**   React positively to and acknowledge patient's and mother's emotions.

☐☐☐ **Fluency**   Speak fluently and do not use jargon.

☐☐☐ **Summarise**   Check with the patient and deliver an appropriate summary.

'Thank you very much for telling me about your son's problems and bringing him today. I understand you are very concerned about his headaches, in particular about the possibility of a brain tumour, and that you would like a computed tomography scan to exclude this. I would like to reassure you, having taken a full history from both you and your son, that I believe it is highly unlikely that James has a brain tumour. Brain tumours are extremely rare in children and in addition to this James's symptoms are highly suggestive of a common migraine. As a result a CT scan would not be indicated or assist the diagnosis.'

EXAMINER'S EVALUATION

1 2 3 4 5
☐☐☐☐☐ Assessment of taking the headache history
☐☐☐☐☐ Role player's score
          Total mark out of 32

DIFFERENTIAL DIAGNOSIS

(See Chapter 3.1.)

3.3   PAEDIATRICS: NEONATAL EXAMINATION

INSTRUCTIONS

You are a foundation year House Officer in paediatrics. Ms Turner delivered a baby boy 12 hours before and now wishes to be discharged. Please carry out an appropriate examination of the neonate and determine whether the newborn may be discharged. Explain to the examiner what you are doing as you proceed.

NOTE

In the OSCE setting you will be provided with a manikin instead of a real neonate. It is important to handle the manikin and examine it with the same respect as if it were a child.

EXAMINATION

1 2 3

☐ ☐ ☐   **Introduction**   Introduce yourself. Establish rapport with the mother.

☐ ☐ ☐   **Request**   Request the maternal obstetric notes. Check blood results, ultrasound scans and general comments.

☐ ☐ ☐   **History**   Take a brief obstetric and birth history from the mother. Establish if there were any maternal illnesses during the pregnancy. Ascertain the type of delivery and whether any anaesthesia or instruments had been used.

Enquire about the condition of the child at birth and the Apgar scores at 1 and 5 minutes. Establish if there were any resuscitative measures used or problems during the birth. Briefly ask if the baby had passed urine (in first 12 hours) and meconium (passed within 48 hours of birth).

Signs	Score of 0	Score of 1	Score of 2
Appearance	Blue	Blue at extremities, pink trunk	Normal pink
Pulse	Absent	< 100 bpm	> 100 bpm
Grimace (reflex irritability)	None	Grimace/feeble cry	Sneeze/cough/pulls away, cries
Activity	None, floppy	Some flexion	Active movement
Respiration	Absent	Weak or irregular	Loud cry

Apgar Score (Out of 10)

The Apgar score is a useful tool that allows an instant assessment of a newborn to determine if he or she requires immediate medical care

| | **Consent** | Explain the examination to the mother and seek consent to perform it. |
| ☐☐☐ | **Wash Hands** | Wash your hands, and undress the baby completely, including removing the nappy. If you are unsure whether the baby will be calm by the end of the examination you may wish to consider auscultating the heart now before he or she becomes restless. |

INSPECTION

| | **General** | Stand at the edge of the bed and observe the baby. Note the baby's appearance, colour, posture, tone, movements and breathing. |
| ☐☐☐ | *Appearance* | Check for dysmorphic features, signs of birth trauma, rashes and baby's size. |

Appearance in the Neonatal Examination

Colour	Jaundice, peripheral cyanosis, pallor, rashes, petechiae (purple spots)
Dysmorphic changes	Dysmorphia, cleft lip, epicanthic folds, single palmar crease, large tongue (Down's syndrome), small jaw and tongue (Pierre–Robin syndrome)
Birth trauma	Caput succedaneum, subconjunctival haemorrhages, moulding, cephalhaematoma, forceps marks
Birth marks	Mongolian blue spots, stork bite, strawberry mark, erythema toxicum, miliaria, congenital melanocytic naevi, café au lait spots
Baby's size	Foetal malnutrition. Weigh the baby and check the weight for length ratio

	Posture	Look for hemiparesis, 'pithed frog' position or opisthotonos (rigidity, arched back, head thrown backwards).
	Tone	Look at the head, arms and legs for generalised hypertonicity (stiff) or hypotonicity (floppy – Down's syndrome).
☐☐☐	*Movements*	Watch limb movements for asymmetrical or abnormal movements (myoclonus, convulsions).
☐☐☐	*Breathing*	Observe the neonate's pattern of breathing, respiratory rate, and chest wall movements and note any added sounds.

Breathing Observations in the Neonatal Examination

Chest shape	Pectus carinatum, pectus excavatum, over-inflation
Pattern of breathing	Regular or irregular
Respiratory rate	Normal (30–50 breaths per minute)
	Dyspnoea (laboured breathing) Tachypnoea (> 60 breaths per minute)
Type of breathing	Periodic apnoea (cessation of breathing for 15–20 seconds)
	Tracheal tug, sub/intercostal recession, nasal flaring, grunting, use of accessory muscles, asymmetrical movements
Additional sounds	Cough, wheeze, stridor (harsh, high/low pitched, continuous)

PALPATION

*Head

☐☐☐ **Fontanelle**   Palpate the anterior and posterior fontanelles, noting if they are depressed and soft (dehydrated) or tense (ICP – hydrocephalus). Start at the frontal bone and follow to the apex of the head. Ascertain if the cranial sutures are fused.

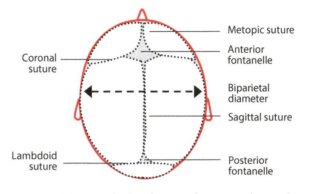

Coronal suture

Lambdoid suture

Metopic suture

Anterior fontanelle

Biparietal diameter

Sagittal suture

Posterior fontanelle

☐☐☐ **Measure**   Measure the head circumference and state that you would like to plot it on a growth centile chart.

Measuring the Head Circumference in a Baby

The head circumference gives an accurate approximation of the volume of the cranial content. It should be measured midway between the child's eyebrows and hairline at the front to the occipital prominence at the back with the tape passing over the ears. An inelastic plastic tape should be employed. The best of several measurements should be documented. The normal-term newborn head circumference is between 33 and 38 cm. Measurements are based on sex and age (weeks, months)

---

*Face

☐☐☐ **Ears**   Note the presence of any ear tags. Draw an imaginary line from the corner of the eye to the ear and establish if the baby has low-set ears (Down's syndrome). Check the patency of the ears and nostrils.

☐☐☐ **Eyes**   Ask for an ophthalmoscope to look for the presence of a red reflex. The absence of a red reflex suggests congenital cataracts, while a white reflex suggests a retinoblastoma. Redness of the sclera could indicate a subconjunctival haemorrhage (birth trauma). Check for abnormal eye movements (squint) and Brushfield spots (Down's syndrome) in the iris.

☐☐☐ **Mouth**   Establish the presence of the rooting reflex by stroking with your finger the corner of the baby's mouth. The baby should turn towards the finger. Insert your finger into the baby's mouth and note if the baby starts to suckle (sucking reflex). Whilst it is in the mouth, raise your finger to palpate the soft palate for a cleft palate (ideally also using a torch for better vision).

*Hands

General Note the presence of palmar creases (Down's syndrome). Count the fingers looking for accessory digits (polydactyly) or fused digits (syndactyly).

*Chest and Heart

☐☐☐ **Capillary Refill** Check for the capillary refill time by placing your thumb on the baby's sternum and noting the time it requires to restore its natural colour. The normal duration is less than 3 seconds.

☐☐☐ **Pulse** Palpate the femoral and brachial pulses sequentially then simultaneously. Note if they are weak, absent or delayed (brachio-femoral delay – coarctation of the aorta). Use the pads of your fingers, avoiding the thumb, when examining for the pulse. A normal heart rate should be 100–160 bpm.

☐☐☐ **Heart** Palpate the praecordium and feel and look for the apex beat. Listen to the heart using the bell of the stethoscope. Listen over the four cardiac areas, similar to an adult, for the presence or absence of murmurs.

☐☐☐ **Lungs** Auscultate the lung fields using the diaphragm of the stethoscope. Listen for asymmetrical air entry, crepitations, rhonchi and bowel sounds.

*Abdomen

General Inspect the abdomen noting the presence of a scaphoid abdomen (diaphragmatic hernia) or a distended abdomen (bowel obstruction) with visible gastric or bowel movements.

☐☐☐ **Umbilicus** Carefully inspect the umbilical stump at the infant's end, counting three umbilical vessels (two arteries and one vein). Look for signs of infection, bleeding or discharge from the stump. The stump should spontaneously separate within a week.

☐☐☐ **Palpation** Palpate the abdomen, in particular the liver (hepatomegaly), spleen (splenomegaly), bladder (outlet obstruction) and masses. Ballot the kidneys to check their presence and size by resting your thumbs in the flank area and your fingers in the loin region.

*Genitalia

☐☐☐ **Boy** Gently palpate the testes, noting if they have descended, and the scrotum for the presence of a hydrocele. If the testes are not in the scrotum, palpate downwards from the inguinal region. Observe for hypospadias (absent urethral orifice, baby urinates via anus).

Girl Make an attempt at separating the vulva, noting for the presence of a vulval fusion, vaginal cysts, tags and discharge.

Hernias Palpate over the inguinal canals for presence of inguinal hernias.

*Hips

☐☐☐ **Special Tests**   Perform Barlow's and Ortolani's test to assess for congenital dislocation of the hip.

Barlow's Test   Perform the Barlow manoeuvre by stabilising the pelvis with the index and middle fingers over the greater trochanter and the thumb over the inner aspect of the infant's thigh. Adduct and flex the hip while applying a gentle downward force in line with the shaft of the femur. In a dislocatable hip, dislocation is felt as a palpable 'clunk' as the femoral head slips out of the acetabulum posteriorly (positive Barlow's sign). The Barlow's manoeuvre tests for an unstable hip that lies in the normal position but can be dislocated.

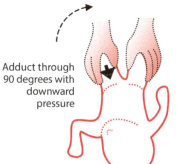

Adduct through 90 degrees with downward pressure

Barlow's Sign

Flex and adduct the baby's hips while applying downward pressure noting for a 'clunk'. Positive sign suggests hip can be dislocated.

Ortolani's Test   Perform the Ortolani's manoeuvre by flexing the baby's hips and knees to 90° with the examiner's thumbs resting on the inner aspect of the infant's thigh, and the index fingers over the greater trochanter. Next gently abduct the hip through 90° feeling for and listening for a distinctive clunk which is palpable and audible as the femoral head is reduced back into the acetabulum. A positive Ortolani's sign indicates the hip is dislocated but reducible. However, a restriction of abduction may suggest an irreducible dislocation.

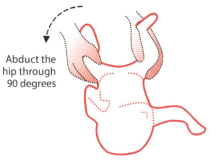

Abduct the hip through 90 degrees

Ortolani's Sign

Flex the baby's hips and knees to 90 degrees and gently abduct the hip through 90 degrees noting for a 'clunk'. Positive sign suggests hip is dislocated.

Significance of the Ortolani's Test

MNEMONIC: ORTOLANI = OUT

Ortolani tests if the hip is **OUT** (dislocated). It is performed by abducting the hip **OUT**wards.

*Feet

☐☐☐   **General**   Inspect the feet, looking for plantar skin creases and clubbed feet (talipes equinovalgus). Count the digits on each foot, checking for accessory digits. Look for calcaneovalgus (abducted forefoot and dorsiflexed ankle). Check full range of movements including dorsiflexion and plantar flexion. Inability to dorsiflex and externally rotate the foot is suggestive of talipes. Turn baby over and now assess the back.

*Back

☐☐☐   **Spine**   Palpate along the spine from the head to the bottom noting any defects (spina bifida occulta, meningomyelocele, meningocele), dermal sinuses or dimples. Look for lipomas, tufts of hair (spina bifida) and port-wine stains.

☐☐☐   **Anus**   Look at the anus and assess if it is patent (anal atresia).

*Posture and Reflexes

☐☐☐   **Head Lag**   Pick up the baby from the supine position by the arms to test for the presence of any head lag.

☐☐☐   **Moro Reflex**   Elicit the Moro reflex by securing the baby's back with the palm of your hand while holding the baby's head with the other hand. Next, release the head by dropping your hand causing it to extend momentarily before supporting it again. The baby will symmetrically abduct, flex and extend his upper limbs. This can be followed by an adduction phase and an audible cry. Asymmetrical movement suggests unilateral paralysis caused by brachial plexus (Erb's palsy, Erb–Duchenne paralysis) or clavicle injury (birth trauma). Bilateral paralysis suggests damage to the central nervous system (brain or spinal cord).

Allow the head to momentarily extend

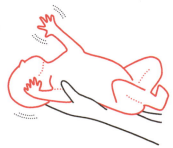

Moro Reflex
Allow the baby's head to suddenly extend. The infant will bilaterally abduct their arms and flex their elbows. Note for a bilateral, unilateral or absent response.

Other Reflexes Elicit the grasp reflex by placing your finger in the baby's palm and observing for finger closure.

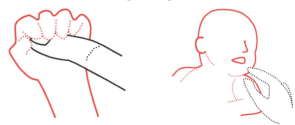

Age Limits for Primitive Reflexes

Plantar grasp	Stroking the baby's palm or sole causes his fingers or toes to grasp. From birth to 4 months. Persistence may suggest a frontal lobe lesion.
Moro reflex	Also known as the startle reflex. It occurs as a response to unexpected loud noise or when the infant feels that he is falling. The child shows a startle response, abducts and then adducts his arms. From birth until 4 months.
Rooting reflex	Associated with the sucking reflex, both reflexes assist breast-feeding. The newborn baby turns his head towards anything that strokes his cheek or mouth. From birth until 4 months.
Tonic neck reflex	The asymmetric tonic neck reflex (ATNR), or parachute reflex, occurs when the child's head is turned to one side, when the ipsilateral arm and leg extend. From birth to 6 months.
Galant's reflex (trunk incurvation)	Hold the baby in ventral suspension and stroke his skin along one side of his back. The baby will swing his trunk and hips to the ipsilateral side being stroked. From birth to 4 months.

☐☐☐ **Weigh** Weigh the child on appropriate paediatric scales and state that you would like to plot the weight on a growth centile chart.

Weight and Height Measurements in a Baby

A baby's growth is best assessed by plotting the baby's height and weight on appropriate charts. Babies should be weighed naked (or with a clean dry nappy) on a self-calibrating or regularly calibrated scale. In an older child, weighing can be performed on a standing scale with minimum clothing. An infant's height should be measured on a calibrated length board. Similarly, babies should be measured naked or with a clean dry nappy. An assistant should hold the baby's head against the headpiece with the head facing upwards. The measurer then brings the footboard gently into contact with the baby's heels with a downward pressure required at the knees to extend both the legs to full length.

Request Tell the family that you would like to perform a heel-prick test (Guthrie test), which tests for phenylketonuria and hypothyroidism, on day 6 of his life.

☐☐☐ **Summarise** Thank the baby's parent. Answer any questions and summarise findings.

Traffic Light System for Identifying Risk of Serious Illness*

Signs or symptoms in the 'red' column are considered as high risk. Symptoms solely in the 'amber' column are recognised as being at intermediate risk. Symptoms and signs only in the 'green' column are deemed low risk.

	Green – low risk	Amber – intermediate risk	Red – high risk
Colour	Normal colour of skin and tongue	Pallor reported	Pale/mottled/blue
Activity	Responds to social cues	Not responding normally to social cues	No response to social cues
	Content/smiles	Wakes only with prolonged stimulation	Appears ill
	Stays awake	Decreased activity	Does not wake
	Strong normal cry	No smile	Weak, continuous cry
Resp.		Nasal flaring, crackles	Grunting, RR > 60 bpm
		RR > 50 bpm, age 6–12 months	Severe or mod. chest indrawing
		RR > 40 bpm, age > 12 months	
		O_2 saturation ≤ 95% in air	
Hydration	Normal skin and eyes	Dry mucous membranes	Reduced skin turgor
	Moist mucous membranes	Poor feeding in infants	
		CRT ≥ 3 seconds	
		Reduced urine output	
Other	No amber or red symptoms	Fever for ≥ 5 days	Age 0–3 months, temp ≥ 38°C
		Swelling of a limb or joint	Age 3–6 months, temp ≥ 39°C
		Non-weight bearing/not using an extremity	Non-blanching rash, bulging fontanelle, neck stiffness, status epilepticus, focal neurological signs
		A new lump > 2 cm	Focal seizures
			Bile-stained vomiting

CRT: Capillary refill time, RR: Respiratory rate.
*Adapted from the NICE guidance on 'Feverish illness in children: Assessment and initial management in children younger than 5 years'

EXAMINER'S EVALUATION

1 2 3 4 5
☐☐☐☐☐ Assessment of the neonate examination
Total mark out of 38

DIFFERENTIAL DIAGNOSIS

Developmental Dysplasia of the Hip (DDH)

Developmental dysplasia of the hip includes a range of developmental hip disorders from mildly dysplastic to severely dysplastic, and dislocated hips. It describes a displacement of the femoral head from the acetabulum disturbing the normal development of the joint. It occurs in 1.5 per 1000 births and is eight times more frequent in girls than in boys. Note that the left hip is twice as often dislocated as the right. This is believed to be due to the foetal position where the baby's left hip rests against the mother's sacrum, thereby restricting its movement. Risk factors include breech birth, first baby, restriction of movement (oligohydramnios) and Down's syndrome. Clinical features include limited abduction of the flexed hip, asymmetry of the inguinal or thigh skin folds, shortening of one leg, positive Ortolani's sign and Barlow's test, abnormal Trendelenburg's test and a waddling gait.

Caput Succedaneum

Caput succedaneum is the accumulation of subcutaneous fluid in the scalp. It is caused by mechanical trauma during childbirth as the presenting portion of the scalp is pushed through the cervix. It is more likely to occur during prolonged labour or vacuum extraction. As opposed to a cephalohaematoma, the effusion overlies the periosteum with poorly defined margins, may cross the midline and over suture lines and consists of serum rather than blood. It is often associated with head moulding. The soft tissue swelling usually resolves over the first few days of life.

Cephalohaematoma

Cephalhaematoma is a subperiosteal collection of blood caused by the rupture of blood vessels between the skull and the periosteum. The bleeding is limited by the suture lines with the parietal region commonly affected. Causes include prolonged labour and instrumental delivery (ventouse, forceps). It presents as a well-demarcated fluctuant swelling that does not cross the suture lines. There is no overlying skin discolouration. It normally appears after 2–3 days of life and takes several weeks to resolve as the blood clot is slowly absorbed from the periphery towards the centre.

Inguinal and Umbilical Hernias

Umbilical hernias are congenital malformations that are common in infants of African descent and more frequent in boys. The incidence of umbilical hernias increases with low birth weight, Down's syndrome and Beckwith–Wiedemann syndrome. They are often asymptomatic and can get quite large in size, but fortunately strangulation is extremely rare. Up to 95% of umbilical hernias spontaneously close within 5 years. A surgical opinion should be sought if a hernia persists for prolonged periods. Inguinal hernias are protrusions of the abdominal cavity contents through the inguinal canal. They are more frequently found in boys (8:1), with the right side (70%) being more common than the left side (25%) and bilateral (5%). They are divided into two categories, direct and indirect hernias. Indirect hernias occur when the abdominal contents herniate through the deep inguinal ring. Direct hernias occur when the abdominal contents protrude and herniate through a weakening in the abdominal wall fascia and into the inguinal canal. They usually present as a painless intermittent lump in the inguinoscrotal region in boys and the inguinolabial region in girls, which increases in size when crying or straining. An inconsolable child with a tender, firm, discoloured lump should be treated with a high suspicion of incarceration.

Undescended Testes

Cryptorchidism is derived from the Greek words *krypto* and *orchis*, which literally mean 'hidden testicle'. It is the absence of one or both testes from the scrotum. However, although cryptorchidism is subtly different from 'undescended testes', the terms are often used interchangeably. Undescended testes are associated with reduced fertility, an increased risk of testicular germ cell tumours and testicular torsions. They are commonly unilateral (66%) but can be bilateral and affect up to 2–3% of male neonates. Most of the time the testis remains palpable along the inguinal canal. However, in a minority of cases the testis is impalpable and resides in the abdomen or is absent. Cryptorchidism can be caused by a congenital absence (anorchia), maldescent or retractile testis (moving between the scrotum and canal). Most descend within the first year of life. Corrective surgery (orchidopexy) should be performed in infancy if the problem persists in order to minimise the risk of complications.

INSTRUCTIONS

This scenario will test your observational skills and ability to make a diagnosis. For this you will need knowledge of developmental milestones and the presentation of certain childhood illnesses. Watch the video closely and complete the questionnaire provided.

DEVELOPMENTAL ASSESSMENT

1 2 3

☐☐☐ **Video** — Observe the video and watch the child playing in their environment.

☐☐☐ **Development** — Assess the four major categories, including fine motor, gross motor, language and social categories (see table).

☐☐☐ **Milestones** — When assessing milestones, consider them in 3-month categories. Determine the child's age by observing for a milestone they can perform within a particular field before assessing for a milestone the child cannot carry out. The child's developmental age will fall within the two limits. It is important to note that the developmental age may not be equal across the four developmental categories. This can be normal for a child.

Age	Fine motor	Gross motor	Language	Social
Birth	Follows face in midline	Symmetrical movements, head lag, flexed posture	Stills to voice Startled by loud noise	Smiles (6 weeks)
3 months	Fixes and follows through 90° (6 weeks), opens hand	Pushes up with arms, head control	Cries, laughs, vocalisation (4 months)	Laughs and squeals
6 months	Reaches, transfers objects, palmar grasp	Sits unsupported	Babbles	Solid food in mouth
9 months	Pincer grasp (9–10 months)	Sits well, pulls to stand	Says Daddy (non-specifically)	Stranger anxiety, plays peek-a-boo
12 months	Mature pincer grasp, releases object	Walks or shuffles	Says Mummy and Daddy (specific)	Waves bye-bye, drinks from cup
18 months	Scribbles, builds 3-cube tower	Adult walk, walks upstairs	5–10 words	Domestic mimicry
2 years	Circular scribbles and lines, builds 6-cube tower	Kicks ball, runs	2-word sentences	Uses spoon and fork, undresses, symbolic and parallel play

Age	Fine motor	Gross motor	Language	Social
3 years	Draws a circle, builds bridge of 3 cubes	Jumps, throws ball, pedal tricycle	Says first and last name, knows colours	Dresses, has friend, interactive play
4 years	Draws a cross or man, builds steps of bricks	Stands on one leg, hops	Counts to 10+	Does buttons, undress
5 years	Draws a triangle	Bicycle, catches ball, skips	Good speech	Ties shoelaces (or good attempt)

☐☐☐ **Age Limits**   Observe for red-flag features that suggest delayed development.

Age Limits for Developmental Milestones

Age	Development sign	Age	Development sign
8 weeks	Smiling, asymmetrical Moro	12 months	Stands upright
3 months	Fixes and follows	12 months	Pincer grip
4 months	Head control (no head lag)	18 months	Walks unsupported
6 months	Reaching out for objects	18 months	Feeds self with spoon
7 months	Polysyllabic babble	30 months	Speaks in phrases
8 months	Transfers	2.5 years	Symbolic play
9 months	Sits unsupported	3.5 years	Interactive play

Motor problems often present early in life (first year) as the child makes an effort to learn how to walk. Language concerns manifest in the second year of life during the period when the child attempts to speak a few words. Behavioural and social issues occur in the third year of life when the child should become more autonomous and interactive.

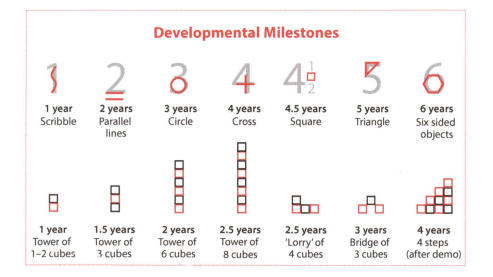

Developmental Milestones

1 year Scribble	**2 years** Parallel lines	**3 years** Circle	**4 years** Cross	**4.5 years** Square	**5 years** Triangle	**6 years** Six sided objects
1 year Tower of 1–2 cubes	**1.5 years** Tower of 3 cubes	**2 years** Tower of 6 cubes	**2.5 years** Tower of 8 cubes	**2.5 years** 'Lorry' of 4 cubes	**3 years** Bridge of 3 cubes	**4 years** 4 steps (after demo)

Milestones in Development of Children

Mnemonic:	1 year	Speaks single words
	2 years	Two-word sentences, understands two-step commands
	3 years	Three-word combinations, repeats three digits, rides tricycle
	4 years	Draws four-sided square, counts four objects

EXAMINER'S EVALUATION

1 2 3 4 5
☐ ☐ ☐ ☐ ☐   Assessment of child development
Total mark out of 13

DIFFERENTIAL DIAGNOSIS

Down's Syndrome (Trisomy 21)

Down's syndrome was first described by John Langdon Haydon Down in 1866. It is one of the most common genetic disorders to cause learning disability in children and affects approximately 1 in 800 births. It is characterised by the presence of an extra copy of genetic material from the 21st chromosome. Up to 95% of children with Down's syndrome obtain the extra chromosome 21 from non-dysjunction at the time of gamete formation. The remaining 5% are the result of either translocation, involving part of the 21st chromosome attaching to another (chromosome 14), or by mosaicism. The incidence of Down's syndrome is strongly associated with maternal age, with the probability of conceiving a 'Down's baby' rapidly increasing after the age of 40 (risk at the age of 30 is 1:900, while at the age of 44 it is 1:37). It is often suspected in children because of a characteristic dysmorphic facial appearance including a round face, epicanthic folds, protruding tongue, Brushfield spots (speckled iris), single palmar creases (simian crease), incurved little finger (clinodactyly), a flat occiput and small stature. Patients also suffer from congenital abnormalities, including cardiac defects (AVSD, VSD, ASD, PDA, tetralogy of Fallot), duodenal atresia, moderate to severe learning disability, atlantoaxial instability and increased risk of chest infections and leukaemias.

Symptoms of Down's Syndrome

MNEMONIC: 'CHILD HAS PROBLEM'

Congenital heart disease (AVSD, VSD, ASD, PDA, T of F), **C**ataracts
Hypotonia, **H**ypothyroidism
Increased gap between 1st and 2nd toe, **I**ncurved little finger (clinodactyly)
Leukaemia risk (increased twofold), **L**ung problems (recurrent chest infections)
Duodenal atresia, **D**ysmorphic facial appearance
Hirschsprung's disease
Atlantoaxial instability, **A**lzheimer's disease
Squint, **S**hort neck
Protruding tongue, **P**almar crease
Round face, **R**olling eye (nystagmus)
Occiput flat, **O**blique eye fissure
Brushfield spots, **B**rachycephaly

Low nasal bridge, **L**anguage problem
Epicanthic fold, **E**ar folded
Mental retardation, **M**yoclonus

Attention Deficit Hyperactivity Disorder (ADHD)

Attention deficit hyperactivity disorder (ADHD), also known as hyperkinetic disorder, is a syndrome diagnosed in approximately 0.1% of British children. It affects boys four times more than girls and is associated with behavioural problems. Features include hyperactivity, poor concentration or inattention, impulsive behaviour, restlessness and becoming easily distracted. Diagnosis is made when symptoms persist for more than 6 months, occur in more than one environment (school, home, shopping) and affect or impair the child's normal function. Symptoms should have an early onset (before the age of 6). Affected children are prone to having often unprovoked temper tantrums and behaving recklessly. The disorder is associated with learning difficulties and is treated under specialist supervision using appropriate drugs (amphetamine or methylphenidate-based) and behavioural therapy.

Autism Spectrum Disorder

Autism is a disorder beginning in early childhood (first 3 years of life) which is associated with impairment of social interaction, communication and abnormal behaviour. Autistic children appear to lack what is widely regarded as normal intuition about the people around them. They exhibit a reduced response to social stimuli (e.g. by not responding to their own name), show reduced social understanding and associated emotional responses (e.g. make poor eye contact and poor use of facial expression). They may also appear to be socially detached individuals, although they do form attachments with their main carers. Impairment of communication normally presents as a delayed onset of cooing or babbling. Later, an inability to articulate useful speech is shown in association with restricted use of non-verbal communication. Autistic children may express an echolalia phenomenon whereby they repeat sounds and words that other people say. They may also ignore grammatical rules in their speech and exhibit pronoun reversals. Abnormal behaviour includes stereotypical movements (hand clapping, hand waving, body swaying), daily ritualistic behaviour and self-injurious behaviour. Autistic children may also exhibit poor imitation of others and a lack of imagination (e.g. during play).

Features of Autism

MNEMONIC: 'AUTISTICS'

Again and again (repetitive behaviour)
Unusual abilities (Asperger's syndrome)
Talking (language) delay
IQ subnormal
Social development poor (less eye contact)
Three years at onset
Inherited component
Communication poor (echolalia)
Self-injurious behaviour

Cerebral Palsy

Cerebral palsy (CP) describes a variety of persistent and non-progressive motor syndromes affecting movement and posture due to disturbances occurring in the foetal or neonatal period. Sensation, cognition and behaviour may also be affected. Although clinical features can depend on the type of cerebral palsy presented, general classical features can include abnormal posture (for example, a slouched posture while sitting), an unsteady gait (including scissoring gait and toe walking), facial gestures (due to involuntary movements) and movements which appear to be clumsy.

3.5 PAEDIATRICS: CARDIOVASCULAR EXAMINATION

INSTRUCTIONS

You are a foundation year House Officer in paediatrics. Examine this child's cardiovascular system. Explain to the examiner what you are doing as you proceed and present a differential diagnosis.

NOTE

When conducting a paediatric examination, it is important to be opportunistic. Be prepared to tailor your examination to the child and be flexible in your approach.

EXAMINATION

1 2 3

☐☐☐ **Introduction** — Introduce yourself. Establish rapport with the child.
Explain — Explain the purpose of the examination and obtain consent from the parent (and child where appropriate) to expose and examine the child.

☐☐☐ **Position** — Sit the child at a 45° angle and expose the patient appropriately. Maintain the child's dignity throughout.

INSPECTION

☐☐☐ **General** — Stand at the edge of the bed and observe the patient. Confirm the child's age and comment on their height and appearance in context of their age. Say that you will check their height and weight on growth charts standardised for age and sex.

General Observations in the Cardiovascular Examination

General health	Nutritional status, failure to thrive
Breathing at rest	Comfortable, dyspnoeic, cough. Check respiratory rate
Colour	Pale, cyanosed (bluish discolouration)
Presence of scars	Midline sternotomy (TGV, valve replacement)
	Left thoracotomy (Blalock–Taussig shunt, PDA ligation, COA repair, pulmonary artery banding)
	Right thoracotomy (Blalock–Taussig shunt, PDA ligation)
Dysmorphic features	Check for features of Down's, Turner's and Marfan's syndrome
Turner's syndrome	Webbed neck, short stature, cubitus valgus (COA, AS)
Down's syndrome	(AVSD, ASD, VSD, tetralogy of Fallot)
Marfan's syndrome	Tall for age, wide arm span and high arched palate (COA, AR, MR, MVP)
Others	Williams syndrome (AS), Noonan's syndrome (PS)

Abbreviations: TGV – transposition of great vessels, VSD – ventricular septal defect, COA coarctation of aorta, ASD – atrial septal defect, AVSD – atrioventricular septal defect, AR/MR – Atrial/mitral regurgitation, MVP – mitral valve prolapse, PDA – patent ductus arteriosus.

□□□ **Hands**   Feel the hands for any temperature change. Look in the hands for:

Hand Signs in the Cardiovascular Examination

Appearance	Arachnodactyly (Marfan's syndrome)
Temperature	Warm and well perfused/poor perfusion (capillary refill normal if < 3 secs)
Peripheral Cyanosis	Blue nail beds
Clubbing	Endocarditis, cyanotic congenital heart disease
Endocarditis (SBE)	Osler nodes and Janeway lesions, splinter haemorrhages

□□□ **Pulse**   In young children the brachial or femoral pulses are easier to palpate and more useful than the radial pulse. Check for the presence of a brachial pulse on either side. Assess the rate, rhythm, volume and character of the right brachial pulse.

Causes of Absent Brachial Pulse

Absent left side	Left Blalock–Taussig shunt, repair of coarctation of aorta
Absent right side	Right Blalock–Taussig shunt
Absent bilaterally	Cardiac catheterisation

□□□ *Rate*   Count for 10 seconds and multiply the rate by six.
Note if it is normal, bradycardic (athletic, heart block, drugs −β-blocker) or tachycardic (anxiety) depending on the normal range for the child's age.

Normal Heart Rates for Healthy Children

Age	Normal range (Beats per minute)
Infant (birth–1 years)	120–160
Toddler (1–3 years)	90–150
Preschool (3–6 years)	80–140
Young children (6–12 years)	70–120
Adolescent (12–18 years)	60–100

□□□ *Rhythm*   Establish the quality of the rhythm. Auscultate at the apex for the apical rate (true heart rate).

Normal Heart Rates for Healthy Children

Regular	Normal healthy children
Regularly irregular	Pulsus bigeminus, extrasystoles
Irregularly irregular	Multiple extrasystoles (common), AF (ASD, surgery, rheumatic MS)

Volume   Establish the pulse volume.

High and Low Pulse Volumes

Low volume	Low cardiac outputs (hypovolaemia), heart failure, aortic stenosis, pericardial effusion
Large volume	Carbon dioxide retention, anaemia, AR, thyrotoxicosis

☐☐☐   *Character*   Assess the character of the pulse.

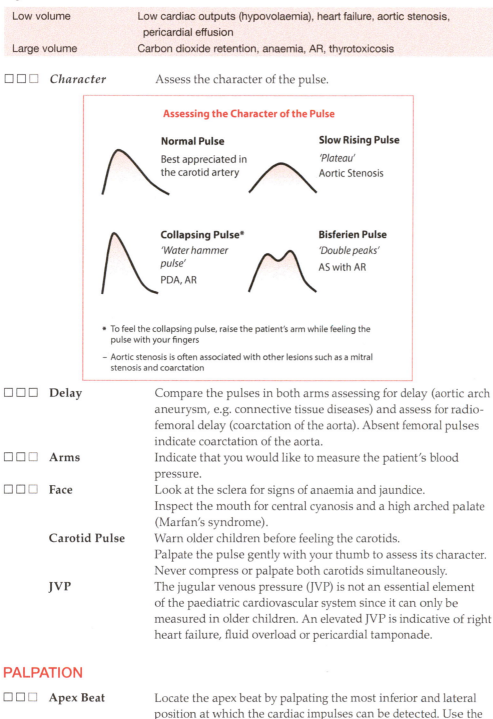

☐☐☐   **Delay**   Compare the pulses in both arms assessing for delay (aortic arch aneurysm, e.g. connective tissue diseases) and assess for radio-femoral delay (coarctation of the aorta). Absent femoral pulses indicate coarctation of the aorta.

☐☐☐   **Arms**   Indicate that you would like to measure the patient's blood pressure.

☐☐☐   **Face**   Look at the sclera for signs of anaemia and jaundice. Inspect the mouth for central cyanosis and a high arched palate (Marfan's syndrome).

      Carotid Pulse   Warn older children before feeling the carotids. Palpate the pulse gently with your thumb to assess its character. Never compress or palpate both carotids simultaneously.

      JVP   The jugular venous pressure (JVP) is not an essential element of the paediatric cardiovascular system since it can only be measured in older children. An elevated JVP is indicative of right heart failure, fluid overload or pericardial tamponade.

PALPATION

☐☐☐   **Apex Beat**   Locate the apex beat by palpating the most inferior and lateral position at which the cardiac impulses can be detected. Use the manubriosternal angle (2nd intercostal space) as well as the mid-clavicular line, anterior and mid-axillary lines as landmarks when describing its location. Above the age of 8 years it is normally located in the 5th intercostal space mid-clavicular line, below 8 years it is in the 4th intercostal space. Note the character of the apex beat and whether it is displaced laterally (left ventricular hypertrophy, pectus excavatum). If it is impalpable, consider dextrocardia or pericardial effusion.

Assessing the Character of the Apex Beat

Tapping	Mitral stenosis
Thrusting	Aortic stenosis
Heaving	Mitral regurgitation, aortic regurgitation
Diffuse	Left ventricular failure, dilated cardiomyopathy

☐☐☐ **Heave and Thrills** Feel for the presence of thrills (palpable murmurs – AS, VSD, PS) by using the flat of the hand to palpate over the praecordium. Use the hypothenar aspect of the hand palpating to the left of the sternum feeling for a parasternal heave (right ventricular hypertrophy).

AUSCULTATION

☐☐☐ **Listen** Auscultate over the four areas of the heart with a stethoscope listening for heart sounds, additional sounds (extra heart sounds, clicks or snaps) and murmurs. Time the murmurs with the right brachial pulse using your thumb to establish if it is a systolic or diastolic murmur.

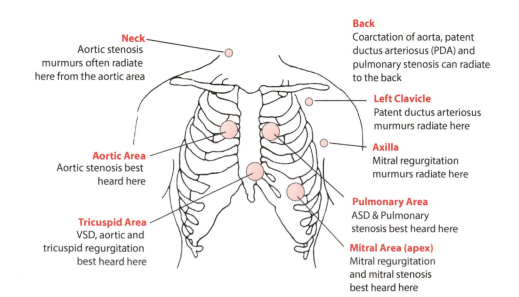

Neck
Aortic stenosis murmurs often radiate here from the aortic area

Back
Coarctation of aorta, patent ductus arteriosus (PDA) and pulmonary stenosis can radiate to the back

Left Clavicle
Patent ductus arteriosus murmurs radiate here

Axilla
Mitral regurgitation murmurs radiate here

Aortic Area
Aortic stenosis best heard here

Tricuspid Area
VSD, aortic and tricuspid regurgitation best heard here

Pulmonary Area
ASD & Pulmonary stenosis best heard here

Mitral Area (apex)
Mitral regurgitation and mitral stenosis best heard here

Auscultation Areas of the Heart

MNEMONIC: 'ALL PATIENTS TAKE MEDS'

Aortic area, **P**ulmonary area, **T**ricuspid area, **M**itral area

Characteristics of Heart Sounds

Loud 1st heart sound	ASD, mechanical prosthetic valve, mitral stenosis
Loud 2nd heart sound	Includes pulmonary flow (PDA, ASD, large VSD), pulmonary hypertension
Soft 2nd heart sound	Tetralogy of Fallot, pulmonary stenosis
Split 2nd heart sound	Normal variation, atrial septal defect (fixed split)
3rd heart sound	Normal variation, left or right ventricular failure
4th heart sound	Left or right ventricular failure, pulmonary hypertension

☐☐☐ *Mitral* Located around the left 5th intercostal space, mid-clavicular line. Listen for mitral stenosis here, using the bell to hear the low-pitched murmur. Ask the patient to hold their breath in expiration, leaning over to the left-hand side. Next listen for mitral regurgitation by using the diaphragm of the stethoscope at the apex. Check for radiation of the murmur to the axilla.

Pulmonary Located around the 2nd intercostal space, left sternal edge. Listen for pulmonary stenosis here using the diaphragm.

☐☐☐ *Aortic* Located around the 2nd intercostal space, right sternal edge. Listen for aortic stenosis in this area. Check for radiation of the murmur to the carotids.

Tricuspid Located around the 5th intercostal space, left sternal edge. Listen for aortic regurgitation by sitting the child forward and asking them to take a deep breath in and out holding it in full expiration no longer than 3 seconds.

Back Remember to listen over the back between the shoulder blades for PS, PDA or COA.

☐☐☐ *Murmurs* Listen for cardiac murmurs noting the timing, intensity, site, character, pitch, radiation and the effect of respiration and position.

Timing Establish if the murmur is systolic, diastolic or continuous in nature.

Systolic, Diastolic and Continuous Murmurs

Systolic	Ejection (AS, PS, ASD), pansystolic (VSD, COA, MR, TR)
Diastolic	Early diastolic (AR, PR), mid-diastolic (MS, TS)
Continuous	Venous hum (innocent murmur), COA, PDA (machinery sound)

Intensity Murmurs are graded in intensity, between one and six.

Grading the Intensity of a Murmur

Grade 1–3 (Thrill absent)	1	Faint and hard to hear with stethoscope
	2	Louder and heard easily with stethoscope
	3	Moderately loud and heard easily with stethoscope
Grade 4–6 (Thrill present)	4	Loud with stethoscope on chest with thrill just palpable
	5	Very loud and easily palpable thrill
	6	Very, very loud and audible without stethoscope

Site	Determine the location on the praecordium where the murmur is best heard. Note if it is best heard in the mitral, pulmonary, aortic or tricuspid area.
Character	Note if the murmur is rumbling (MS), blowing (MR) or harsh (AS) in character. Assess if it is a crescendo-decrescendo, decrescendo, crescendo or plateau type of murmur.
Pitch	Assess the pitch of the murmur. High-pitched murmurs are best heard with the diaphragm (AS) while low-pitched murmurs are best heard with the bell (MS).
Radiation	Check if the murmur radiates to the carotids (AS), axilla (MR), left sternal edge (AR) or to the back (PDA, PS and coarctation of aorta).
Respiration	Mnemonic for the effect of respiration on murmurs: **RILE** – **R**ight-sided murmurs are heard with greatest intensity in **I**nspiration while **L**eft-sided murmurs are heard with greatest intensity in **E**xpiration.
Position	Note if the murmur is best heard in the supine position (most murmurs), leaning forward with breath held in exhalation (AR) or in the left lateral position (MR).

Signs and Symptoms of Innocent Murmurs

THE MNEMONIC OF MULTIPLE SS

The **S**ymptom-less patient that has a **S**ystolic murmur in a **S**mall area (**S**ite), which is **S**hort in duration, **S**oft in sound with a possible **S**plit **S**econd heart sound. There are no **S**igns present with normal **S**pecial tests (ECG, X-ray, echo).

☐☐☐ **Lung Bases**	Keep the patient leaning forwards and auscultate the lung bases listening for crepitations and pleural effusion (heart failure).
☐☐☐ **Oedema**	Examine for sacral oedema by applying firm pressure for at least 15 seconds against the lower back and for pedal oedema by pressing down over the distal shaft of the tibia. Observe pitting oedema by looking for an indentation of your finger after applying pressure. Ensure that you ask the child if they feel any pain when being pressed.

Liver	Lie the child flat and palpate and percuss for hepatomegaly (heart failure).

Characteristic Features of Heart Failure

Symptoms	Breathlessness on feeding or exertion, sweating, poor feeding and weight gain, recurrent chest infections
Signs	Tachypnoea, tachycardia, galloping rhythm, heart murmur, sweating, cool peripheries, failure to thrive, cardiomegaly, hepatomegaly
Investigations	X-ray (cardiomegaly), ECG, echo (congenital heart disease)

ADDITIONAL POINTS

□□□	**Pulses**	Palpate the peripheral pulses (femoral, popliteal, post tibial, dorsalis pedis).
	Request	Ask to measure the blood pressure, take an ECG tracing and a chest X-ray of the patient. Mention that you would like to have a look at the patient's oxygen saturations and temperature chart.
□□□	**Summarise**	Check with the patient and deliver an appropriate summary.

EXAMINER'S EVALUATION

1 2 3 4 5
□□□□□ Assessment of cardiovascular system
□□□□□ Role player's score
Total mark out of 36

DIFFERENTIAL DIAGNOSIS

Pathology	Pulse rate	Pulse character	Apex	Systolic/ Diastolic	S1	S2
Aortic stenosis	Reg	**Slow-rising	Thrusting **Displaced	Ejection systolic	N	**Quiet
VSD	Normal	Normal/ **collapsing	Normal	Pansystolic 'HARSH'	N	N
PDA	Normal	Collapsing	Normal	Continuous machinery	N	N
Dextrocardia	Normal	Normal	Right 4th intercostal space, Mid-clavic line	No murmurs	N	N

Position	Radiation	Other associations	Diagram	Notes
2nd ICS R sternal edge in expiration	Carotids	**Reversed splitting S2 Gets louder with Valsava **Progressively later peak of murmur in systole	S1 — Soft S2 — **EC** – Ejection click	5% of congenital defects. Associated with mitra stenosis and coarctation of the aorta.
4th ICS L sternal edge Expiration or inspiration (depending on shunt)	Liver	Maladie de Roger: the loudness of the murmur bears no relation to severity of defect Eisenmenger's: reversal to R>L Pulmonary hypertension	S1 — A2 P2 Loud — Pansystolic murmur	Common – represents 30% of newborn heart defects – association with Down's, Edwards and Patau's syndromes.
Mid-scapula region on back	Back	Bears no relation to the cardiac cycle May progress to heart failure (high output)	S1 — A2 P2 — Continuous murmur	Shunt between pulmonary artery and aorta
Auscultation occurs in right chest with non-deviated trachea	Nil	See notes	Nil	Observe for associated features – situs inversus, sinusitus, bronchiectus = Kartagener's – nasal polyps, hearing loss and infertility also occur.

Pathology	Pulse rate	Pulse character	Apex	Systolic/ Diastolic	S1	S2
Atrial septal defect	Normal	Normal – may be bounding in Eisenmenger	Non-displaced	Ejection systolic murmur	N	fixed split
Pulmonary stenosis	Normal	Normal if isolated – may accompany other defects	Non-displaced. Parasternal heave.	Ejection systolic murmur	N	Loud with click – soft if severe
Coarctation of aorta	Radio-femoral delay	N	N	Ejection systolic murmur	N	May be quiet if with AS
Fallot's tetralogy	N	Bounding in Eisenmengers	N	VSD, pulmonary stenosis and right ventricular hypertrophy	N	Single second heart sound

Position	Radiation	Other associations	Diagram	Notes
Loudest in pulmonary region	To pulmonary area	The murmur heard is a pulmonary flow murmur.	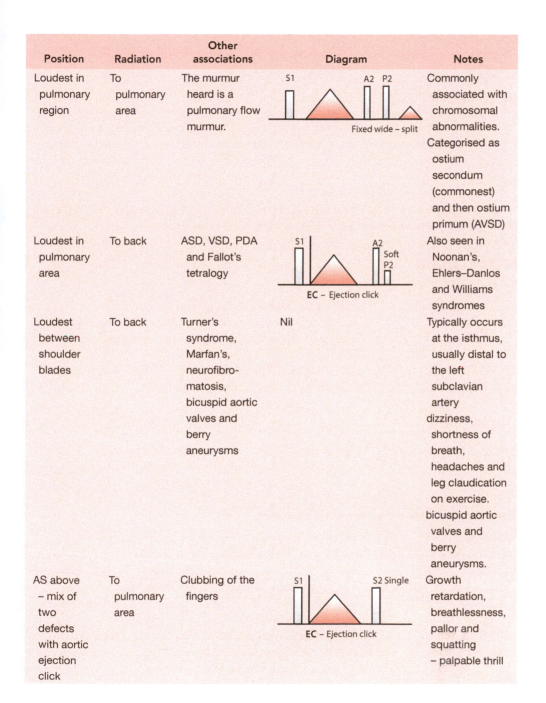	Commonly associated with chromosomal abnormalities. Categorised as ostium secundum (commonest) and then ostium primum (AVSD)
Loudest in pulmonary area	To back	ASD, VSD, PDA and Fallot's tetralogy		Also seen in Noonan's, Ehlers–Danlos and Williams syndromes
Loudest between shoulder blades	To back	Turner's syndrome, Marfan's, neurofibromatosis, bicuspid aortic valves and berry aneurysms	Nil	Typically occurs at the isthmus, usually distal to the left subclavian artery dizziness, shortness of breath, headaches and leg claudication on exercise. bicuspid aortic valves and berry aneurysms.
AS above – mix of two defects with aortic ejection click	To pulmonary area	Clubbing of the fingers		Growth retardation, breathlessness, pallor and squatting – palpable thrill

3.6   PAEDIATRICS: RESPIRATORY EXAMINATION

INSTRUCTIONS

You are a foundation year House Officer in paediatrics. Examine this child's respiratory system. Explain to the examiner what you are doing as you proceed and present a differential diagnosis.

NOTE

When conducting a paediatric examination, it is important to be opportunistic. Be prepared to tailor your examination to the child and be flexible in your approach.

EXAMINATION

1 2 3

☐ ☐ ☐   **Introduction**   Introduce yourself. Establish rapport with the child.
          Explain   Explain the purpose of examination and obtain consent from the parent (and child where appropriate) to expose and examine the child.

☐ ☐ ☐   **Position**   Sit the child at a 45° angle and expose the patient appropriately. Maintain the child's dignity throughout.

INSPECTION

☐ ☐ ☐   **General**   Stand at the edge of the bed and observe the patient. Look for oxygen masks, nebulisers, peak flow meters and sputum pots surrounding the patient.

General Observations in the Respiratory Examination

Development	Height and weight for age (offer to check this against a growth chart)
Breathing at rest	Dyspnoea, pursed lips, nasal flaring, grunting, tracheal tug
Added sounds	Coughing, wheezing, stridor, barking cough (croup)
Chest shape	Barrel chest (air trapping), pectus excavatum (sunken sternum), pectus carinatum (pigeon chest – chronic airway obstruction), Harrison's sulcus (diaphragm insertion – asthma)
Chest movements	Asymmetrical expansion, accessory muscles, sub/intercostal recession
Skin, scars, misc.	Eczema (atopic), engorged superficial veins (SVC obs), thoracotomy scar, operative scars, gastrostomy, portacath, chest drain

☐ ☐ ☐   *Rate*   Count the respiratory rate for 10 seconds and multiply it by six. Note if it is normal, tachypnoeic or dyspnoeic in nature.

Normal Respiratory Rates for Healthy Children

Age	Normal range (Breaths per minute)
Infant (birth–1 year)	30–60
Toddler (1–3 years)	20–30
Preschool (3–6 years)	22–34
Young children (6–12 years)	18–30
Adolescent (> 12 years)	12–16

☐☐☐   **Hands**   Feel the hands for any temperature change. Look at the hands for:

Hand Signs in the Respiratory Examination

Temperature	Warm and well perfused/poor perfusion
Tremor	Resting tremor (beta agonist – salbutamol)
Peripheral cyanosis	Blue nail beds
Clubbing	Bronchiectasis, cystic fibrosis

Pulse   Feel the radial pulse (in small children the brachial) and assess the rate and rhythm. Assess for the presence of a bounding pulse (CO_2 retention).

☐☐☐   **Arms**   Indicate that you would like to measure the patient's blood pressure.

☐☐☐   **Face and Neck**   Look at the conjunctiva for signs of anaemia. Inspect the mouth for central cyanosis. Examine the jugular venous pressure (only in older children) between the two heads of the sternocleidomastoid muscle.

PALPATION

☐☐☐   **Lymph Nodes**   Observe for any enlarged lymph nodes. Sit the patient forward and palpate the lymph nodes in the cervical region and supraclavicular fossa.

Trachea   Palpate the tracheal position by placing the index and middle finger on either side of the trachea. Be gentle and warn the child that it may feel uncomfortable. Determine if it is central or deviated to one side.

☐☐☐   **Apex Beat**   Palpate the apex beat by feeling the furthest pulsating point of the heart. It is normally located in the 4th or 5th (depending on age) intercostal space mid-clavicular line. Determine if the apex beat is displaced (effusion, tension pneumothorax, collapse).

☐☐☐   **Expansion**   Assess chest expansion by placing your hands on the patient's chest with the thumbs just touching in the midline and fingers spread along the ribcage. Ask the patient to breathe normally and then to take deep breaths in. Measure the distance between your thumbs. Note if chest expansion is bilaterally or unilaterally reduced.

PERCUSSION

☐☐☐ **Chest** Place the middle finger of one hand on the patient's chest wall and percuss the centre of the middle phalanx with the middle finger of the other. Percuss the upper, middle and lower zones including the apex, lateral areas and axilla, comparing the percussion note on both sides.

Character of Percussion Note

Stony dull	Pleural effusion
Dull	Consolidation, lung collapse, fibrosis
Resonant	Normal lung
Hyper-resonant	Pneumothorax, air trapping (asthma)

AUSCULTATION

☐☐☐ **Chest** With the child relaxed, request them to breathe deeply through their mouth demonstrating how to do so if necessary. Use the bell of your stethoscope to listen to the apices of the lung and then the diaphragm to listen over the different lung areas mentioned above for breath sounds (bronchial breathing, vesicular breathing, present or absent) or added sounds (wheezes, crackles).

Breath Sounds (BS) on Auscultation

Vesicular breathing	Inspiration followed by expiration without interruption (normal)
Bronchial breathing	Audible gap between inspiratory and expiratory (consolidation, fibrosis)
Reduced BS	ARDS, asthma, pleural effusion, pneumothorax, collapse
Increased BS	Consolidation
Prolonged expiration	Asthma, emphysema
Added sounds	Check for the presence of wheezes, crackles or a pleural rub
Wheezes (rhonchi)	Asthma, pulmonary oedema, HF
Crackles (crepitations)	ARDS, bronchiectasis, consolidation, pulmonary oedema, early HF
Pleural rub	Pneumonia, pneumothorax

☐☐☐ **Vocal Resonance** If the child is mature enough to follow commands, assess vocal resonance by asking the patient to say 'ninety-nine' while listening over the lung areas.
Sit the patient forward and repeat the chest expansion, percussion and auscultation on the back.

Differentials for Stridor

MNEMONIC: 'ABCDEFGH'

Fever	**A**bscess, **B**acterial tracheitis, **C**roup, **D**iphtheria, **E**piglottitis
Without fever	**F**oreign body, **G**as (toxic gas), **H**ypersensitivity

ADDITIONAL POINTS

☐☐☐ **Oedema**   Examine for sacral oedema by applying firm pressure for at least
15 seconds over the sacrum and, for ankle oedema, by pressing
down over the distal shaft of the tibia. Observe pitting oedema
by looking and feeling for an indentation of your finger after
applying pressure. Ensure that you ask the patient if they feel
any pain while you are pressing them.

☐☐☐ **Request**   Ask to take a peak flow (and chest X-ray) of the patient. Say that
you would like to have a look at the patient's oxygen saturations
and temperature chart. Send any abnormally coloured sputum
for microbiology (Gram and ZN stain), culture and cytology.

Different Colours of Sputum

Green: (acute) pneumonia, abscess (chronic) COPD, bronchiectasis. Ask if it has changed.
Yellow: suppurative diseases as above
Black: asbestosis
Rusty-gold: said to be typical of pneumococcal pneumonia
Blood-stained: haemoptysis – think PE, TB, Goodpasture's
Pink, frothy: pulmonary oedema

☐☐☐ **Summarise**   Check with the patient and deliver an appropriate summary.

EXAMINER'S EVALUATION

1 2 3 4 5
☐☐☐☐☐ Assessment of respiratory system
☐☐☐☐☐ Role player's score
         Total mark out of 30

DIFFERENTIAL DIAGNOSIS

Diagnosis	Symptoms	Management
Cystic fibrosis	1 in 2500 carrier rate of 1 in 25 and is more common in Caucasians. CTFR gene on chromosome 7 commonest defect. Recurrent chest infections, failure to thrive, bronchiectasis, pneumothorax, sinusitis and aspergilosis. Look for ports – Port-a-Cath for longterm abx access, PEG for (catheter port) – emerging from the gastric area for additional overnight feeds to maintain nutrition. Finger clubbing, hyperinflated chest with coarse creps, evident expiratory rhonchi and nasal polyps. (See below for mnemonic.)	Sweat test and genetic testing Conservative measures – regular chest physiotherapy, management of bronchiectasis exarbations, maintain nutrition Antibiotics – indicated for flares and role in preventative measures Surgery – isolated lobectomy, double lung transplant often needed later in life, pancreatic transplant
Asthma	Diurnal variation in symptoms, dry cough, wheeze (not always present) – exposure to irritants (dust, smoke) may reflect in pattern of symptoms – e.g better on the weekend. Commonly associated with eczema, allergies and positive family history. Hyperinflated chest with prolonged expiratory phase, pectus carinatum and Harrison's sulci, eczema (atopy), a generalised expiratory wheeze, tachypnoea, intercostal recessions and accessory muscle usage.	Avoid smoking at home – including changing clothes (significant risk with smoke particles in clothing) Routine treatment bronchodilators May require preventative inhalers (see NICE guidance) Acute exarcerbation – check severity of illness. Seek help early and follow protocol escalation of bronchodilators.
Bronchiolitis	Usually caused by a viral infection of the bronchioles – respiratory syncytial virus (RSV) is implicated in 70% of cases. Other causes include adenovirus, influenza and the parainfluenza virus. Predominantly seen in the winter months (from November to February). Symptoms include coryza preceding a cough, a low-grade fever, increasing shortness of breath, an audible wheeze, irritability and poor feeding. On examination, intercostal and subcostal recession, hyperinflated chest, widespread fine inspiratory crepitations and high-pitched wheeze can be ascertained.	May require management in hospital if signs of severe respiratory distress or requiring additional oxygen.

Diagnosis	Symptoms	Management
Croup (laryngo-tracheobronchitis)	Usually caused by parainfluenza virus but RSV, adenovirus and influenza virus. 3 months to 3 years with peak incidence at 2 years of age. Symptoms are generated by the narrowing of the airway, particularly of the larynx, trachea and bronchi. Symptoms include a harsh barking cough (or seal-like bark which is pathognomonic), inspiratory stridor and hoarseness preceding a low-grade fever and coryza (**mnemonic** of croup symptoms: **Three S's** – Stridor, Subglottic swelling, Seal-bark cough). Worse at night. Moderate and severe symptoms include sternal and suprasternal recession at rest, inspiratory and expiratory stridor, respiratory distress, agitation and drowsiness.	An AP film can be performed to reveal the steeple sign (narrowing of the subglottic lumen by 1–1.5 cm producing an inverted 'V' configuration resembling a church's steeple). Croup should be differentiated from epiglottitis, which is a life-threatening emergency due to respiratory obstruction.
Pneumonia	Maybe bacterial, viral or parasitic infection of the lung. Symptoms include fever, cough, lethargy, poor feeding, pleuritic chest pain and shortness of breath. Signs: reduced breath sounds over the affected area, dullness to percussion, bronchial breathing with increased vocal fremitus and crepitations on auscultation.	A chest X-ray may reveal evidence of consolidation and a sputum or blood culture may disclose the causative organism.

Features of Cystic Fibrosis

MNEMONIC: 'CF PANCREAS'

Cough (chronic)
Failure to thrive
Pancreatic insufficiency
Appetite decrease
Nasal polyps
Clubbing, **C**hest infections
Rectal prolapse
Electrolyte elevation in sweat, salty skin
Atresia of vas deferens (infertility)
Sputum (Staphylococcus, Pseudomonas)

Features of Severe and Life-threatening Asthma

Acute severe	Child too breathless to speak or feed
	Respiratory rate > 40 breaths per minute in children 1–5, > 30 breaths per minute in children > 5
	Heart rate > 140 beats per minute in children 1–5, > 125 beats per minute in children > 5
	Peak flow 33–50% of best predicted value
Life-threatening	Agitated (hypoxia) or reduced levels of consciousness (hypercapnia)
	Fatigued or exhausted
	Silent chest, cyanosed or poor respiratory effort
	Peak flow < 33% of best predicted value

Croup

Differentiating between Croup and Epiglottitis

Epiglottitis	Croup
Affects (usually) 1 to 6 years of age	Affects (usually) 3 months to 3 years of age
Rapid onset (hours)	Slow onset (days)
Absent or weak cough	Barking (seal-like) cough
No preceding coryza	Preceding coryza
Drooling saliva	Able to swallow
Temperature > 38.5°C	Temperature < 38.5°C
Weak, whispering voice	Hoarse voice
Unable to eat or drink (painful throat)	Able to eat and drink
Soft continuous stridor, unwilling to speak	Harsh inspiratory stridor
Toxic, upright, mouth open, immobile	Appears unwell but communicative

Pneumonia

Causative Organisms of Pneumonia in Children

Newborn	Group B beta haemolytic
	Streptococcus Escherichia coli (E. coli)
	Gram-negative bacilli
	Chlamydia trachomatis
Infancy	Respiratory syncytial virus (RSV)
	Streptococcus pneumoniae
	Haemophilus influenzae
	Staphylococcus aureus
Older children	Mycoplasma pneumoniae
All ages	Tuberculosis

3.7   PAEDIATRICS: ABDOMEN EXAMINATION

INSTRUCTIONS

You are a foundation year House Officer in paediatrics. Examine this child's abdominal system. Explain to the examiner what you are doing as you proceed and present your differential diagnosis.

NOTE

When conducting a paediatric examination, it is important to be opportunistic. Be prepared to tailor your examination to the child and be flexible in your approach.

EXAMINATION

1 2 3

☐☐☐ **Introduction**   Introduce yourself. Establish rapport with the child.
        Explain   Explain the purpose of the examination and obtain consent from the parent (and child where appropriate) to expose and examine the child.

☐☐☐ **Position**   Lie the patient flat on the couch and expose the abdomen by lowering the child's clothes to the pubic symphysis.

INSPECTION

☐☐☐ **General**   Observe the patient from the edge of the bed. Check if the child's physical appearance is consistent with their age and comment on their nutritional status. Note the shape of the abdomen, evidence of distension or abnormal movements. Inspect for any visible organomegaly or any masses, commenting on site, size, overlying discolouration and cough impulse.

General Observations in the Abdomen Examination

Development	Height and weight for age (check against growth chart)
Stoma sites	Ileostomy, colostomy, gastrostomy, nephrostomy
Catheters/tubes	Nasogastric tube, central line (TPN), continuous ambulatory peritoneal dialysis or other dialysis catheters
Abdominal contour	Flat, scaphoid (sunken), protuberant (normal – young children)
Presence of scars	Roll the child onto their side in order to avoid missing any scars located on the back
Abdominal movements	Gastric peristalsis (pyloric stenosis, intestinal obstruction) or pulsations
Distension	Ascites (umbilical eversion), intestinal obstruction, faeces, hernias
Wasted buttocks	Coeliac disease (weight loss)

☐☐☐ **Hands**   Feel the hands and inspect the nails. Look in the hands for:

Hand Signs in the Abdomen Examination

Clubbing	IBD, coeliac disease, biliary cirrhosis and billiary atresia
	Chronic active hepatitis, CF
Palmar erythema	Chronic liver disease
Leuconychia	Cirrhosis
Koilonychia	Iron deficiency (coeliac disease)

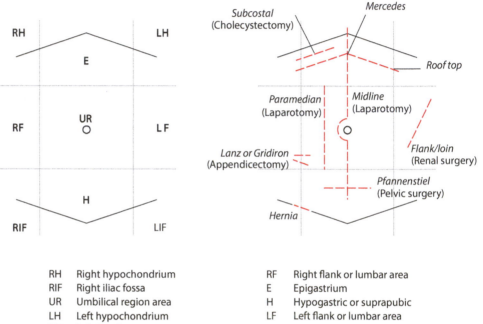

RH	Right hypochondrium		RF	Right flank or lumbar area
RIF	Right iliac fossa		E	Epigastrium
UR	Umbilical region area		H	Hypogastric or suprapubic
LH	Left hypochondrium		LF	Left flank or lumbar area
LIF	Left iliac fossa			

☐☐☐ **Face**   With patient looking down, lift one eyelid and look at the sclera for signs of jaundice and anaemia. Kayser–Fleischer rings in the periphery of the cornea appear in children with Wilson's disease, best seen under slitlamp examination. Look around the lips for brown freckles (Peutz–Jeghers syndrome). Inspect the mouth for:

Signs in the Tongue in the Abdomen Examination

Central cyanosis	Blue tongue
Macroglossis	Congenital hypothyroidism, Beckwith–Wiedemann syndrome
Atrophic glossitis	Iron, folate, B12 deficiency
Dry tongue	Dehydration
Ulcers	Crohn's, coeliac disease, Behcet's disease
Breath smell	Ketosis, foetor hepaticus

Body   Inspect the rest of the body for skin changes and visible manifestation of hepatic impairment including bruising, petechiae, spider naevi and caput medusa (dilated collateral veins around umbilicus).

PALPATION

☐☐☐   **Abdomen**

Enquire if the child has any tenderness in their abdomen by asking: 'Does your tummy hurt?' Explain to the youngster in simple terms what you intend to do. If the child is young you may wish to demonstrate on a toy how you will be palpating his abdomen. Be cautious not to be patronising when talking to an adolescent.

Distraction Techniques when Examining a Child

1   Play 'peek-a-boo' or blow 'raspberries' at infants
2   Permit toddlers to play with your instruments (stethoscope, ophthalmoscope)
3   Provide infants with something to hold (their favourite toy)
4   Engage them in conversation (discuss computer games, school, best friends)

Warm your hands and examine the child at their level by kneeling down. Look at the child's face for grimacing while palpating for signs of local tenderness. A toddler may initially resist you examining them. Employ distraction techniques if necessary. If unsuccessful, use the child's hand to guide yours around his abdomen.

☐☐☐   *Light Palpation*

Palpate all quadrants of the abdomen starting away from the site of the pain. Note any tenderness, rebound tenderness (greater pain felt on releasing pressure), guarding (reflex contraction of abdominal muscles) or rigidity.

Deep Palpation

Palpate all quadrants more deeply. Feel for masses and deep tenderness. If a mass is detected, note its size, shape, edge, consistency, percussion note and the presence of bowel sounds or a thrill.

☐☐☐   **Liver**

Palpate the liver from the right iliac fossa. Ask the child to take deep breaths in. During inspiration, press firmly inwards and upwards using the flat of your hand to palpate the liver. Allow the liver edge to slip under your fingertips as the liver descends. Progressively palpate towards the costal margin.

Feel for an enlarged liver describing its edge (smooth, irregular), size (in centimetres below costal margin), consistency (soft, firm, hard), nodularity and tenderness.

Causes of Hepatomegaly

The liver edge can be normally found 1–2 cm below the costal margin. However, the anterior border is hidden beneath the ribs but can be determined by percussion. It enlarges towards the RIF and moves with respiration

Infection	Hepatitis A B C, infectious mononucleosis, malaria
Malignancy	Leukaemia, lymphoma, neuroblastoma
Liver disease	Neonatal liver disease, chronic liver disease, polycystic disease
Metabolic	Reye's syndrome, glycogen storage disorders, galactosaemia, Wilson's disease, alpha-1 antitrypsin deficiency
Haematological	Haemolytic disease of newborn (sickle cell disease, thalassaemia)
Congestion	Heart failure, biliary atresia

□□□ **Spleen**   Palpate the spleen from the right iliac fossa towards the left hypochondrium using the same technique for the liver edge. The spleen should be found between the 9th and 11th ribs extending to the anterior axillary line in adolescents, but in infancy it can be felt on inspiration as a soft swelling as far as 1–2 cm below the costal margin. Feel for a notch, size, consistency and tenderness.

Causes of Splenomegaly

The spleen can normally be felt just below the costal margin. It has a smooth soft edge posteriorly with the anterior border hidden beneath the ribs. The spleen moves with respiration. During infancy, a 1–2 cm spleen tip is usually palpable

Infective	Malaria (massive splenomegaly, fever and rigors), SBE, infective endocarditis, typhoid, infectious mononucleosis, TB (fever, weight loss, CNS signs), toxoplasmosis
Haematological	Sickle cell disease
Malignancy	Leukaemia (massive), lymphoma (lymphadenopathy, weight loss, CNS signs)
Congestion	Portal hypertension (portal vein obstruction, cirrhosis)

□□□ **Kidneys**   Ballot the kidneys on inspiration. Position one hand beneath the patient's lower rib cage and the other hand on the surface of the abdomen. Ask the patient to breath in deeply. Attempt to push the kidney with the lower hand onto the finger tips of the resting hand. Note any tenderness or enlargement.

Causes of Enlarged Kidneys

The kidneys are usually not palpable after the neonatal period. They can be palpated by balloting bimanually. They also move with respiration

Unilateral enlarged Polycystic kidney disease, perinephric abscess, hydronephrosis, malignant (hypernephroma, nephroblastoma)

Bilateral enlarged Polycystic kidney disease, hydronephrosis, nephroblastoma

PERCUSSION

☐☐☐ **Liver** Inform the child that you wish to percuss their abdomen 'like a drum'. Percuss the upper and lower liver borders to detect any enlargement. Note a change in percussion note from resonant to dull. The normal liver span varies with height and sex but is generally located between the 4th and 6th rib (mid-clavicular line) and the costal margin or up to 1–2 cm below the costal margin in children aged up to 3 years. The upper limit of normal for the liver span is 8 cm at 5 years and 13 cm by puberty onwards.

Causes of Hepatosplenomegaly

Hepatosplenomegaly is the concurrent enlargement of both the spleen and liver. There are usually other associated signs to support your diagnosis

Infective Malaria, SBE, infectious mononucleosis

Haematological Sickle cell disease, thalassaemia

Congestion Portal hypertension (portal vein obstruction, cirrhosis)

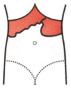

☐☐☐ **Spleen** Percuss the spleen employing a similar technique as for the liver.

Differentiating Between the Left Kidney and an Enlarged Spleen

Splenomegaly	Left kidney
Palpable in infants (not in older children)	Usually not palpable (after birth)
Notched edge	Smooth shape
Moves early in inspiration	Moves late in inspiration
Dull to percussion in Traub's space	Resonant to percussion
Cannot get above the spleen (ribs on top)	Possible to get above the kidney
Not ballotable	Manually ballotable
Enlarges towards RIF in older children but LIF in infants	Directed downwards

☐☐☐ **Ascites** Examine the child for shifting dullness or fluid thrill.
Shifting Dullness Percuss from the umbilicus towards the flanks while noting the point of dullness. Roll the child towards you keeping your finger over this point. Wait 30 seconds and percuss the marked point again to see if the dullness has shifted. Return the patient to the supine position and check if dullness has returned to this point.

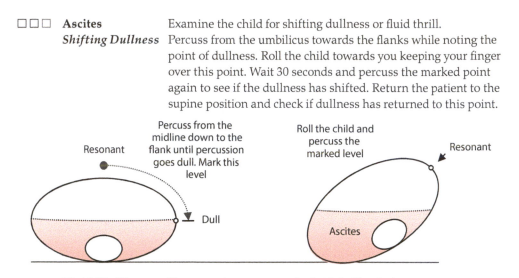

Fluid Thrill To assess the presence of a fluid thrill, ask the young person or parent for assistance. Place the assistant's hand along the midline of the child's abdomen. Place your detecting hand in the flank area while softly flicking the surface of the skin on the opposite flank area with your index finger. The presence of a fluid thrill suggests severe ascites.

☐☐☐ **Bladder** Percuss the suprapubic area for dullness (bladder distension).

AUSCULTATION

☐☐☐ **General** Listen over the abdomen with a stethoscope for peristaltic bowel sounds. Listen for 30 seconds and establish the number of sounds heard (at least 2–3 in 30 seconds). Determine if they are hyperactive ('tinkling' – obstruction), hypoactive or absent (general peritonitis, paralytic ileus).

Renal Bruits Listen over the renal arteries, approximately 2–3 cm superior and lateral to the umbilicus, for bruits (renal artery stenosis).

ADDITIONAL POINTS

☐☐☐ **Hernias** Feel for a cough impulse over the hernial orifices as the patient coughs.

Nodes Feel for inguinal lymph nodes.

☐☐☐ **Request** For the purpose of completion, state that you would like to examine the external genitalia, inguinal and perianal regions, including a PR examination. However, you would not be expected to do this in the OSCE as it is likely to upset the child. Request to dipstick the urine.

☐☐☐ **Summarise** Check with the patient and deliver an appropriate summary.

EXAMINER'S EVALUATION

1 2 3 4 5
☐☐☐☐☐ Assessment of abdomen examination
☐☐☐☐☐ Role player's score
Total mark out of 32

DIFFERENTIAL DIAGNOSIS

Diagnosis	Symptoms	Management
Coeliac disease	Classically – steatorrhoea, weight loss and pallor. Failure to thrive, constipation and abdominal distension. Gluten-sensitive enteropathy > villous atrophy > malabsorption. 1 in 2000 in the UK, but higher in Ireland 1 in 300. Presents in children between 6–24 months.	Primary management is a gluten-free diet. Autoantibody screen followed by on-gluten small bowel biopsy to confirm diagnosis. Specialist paediatric management for assessment.
Inflammatory bowel disease	Spectrum of disease: Crohn's colitis, ileitis and ulcerative colitis. 25% of patients with IBD present as children. Crohn's: mouth to anus affected, perianal disease common. Ulcerative colitis: continous colonic involvement. Assoc: uveitis, erythema nodosum and arthritis.	Large bowel biopsy: transmural inflammation, skip lesions, ulcers and ileitis = Crohn's. Partial inflammation, continuous inflammation – and absence of vascular markings = UC. Induce remission – may require hospitalisation = surgery for steroids and immunosuppressants. Maintain remission – long-term immunosuppression
Kidney transplant	Commonest cause of chronic renal failure is structural malformation – vesicoureteral reflux from posterior urethral valves, pelviureteric or vesicoureteric junction obstruction). Chronic glomerulnehpritis and tubulointerstitial disease, cystic renal disease, haemolytic-uraemic syndrome and heriditary nephropathies less common. Polycystic kidney disease autosomal recessive – presents in infancy. (Autosomal dominant type) does *not* present in childhood. Typically transplant small right iliac fossa mass.	Long-term immunosuppression Surveillance for increased lifetime risk of melanoma and other cancers is very important.

Features of Crohn's disease

MNEMONIC: 'CHRISTMAS'

Cobblestones on endoscopy
High temp (fever)
Reduced lumen
Intestinal fistulae
Skip lesions
Transmural (all layers, aphthous muscles)
Malabsorption
Abdominal pain
Submucosal fibrosis

3.8   PAEDIATRICS: GAIT AND NEUROLOGICAL FUNCTION

INSTRUCTIONS

You are a foundation year House Officer in paediatrics. Examine this child's gait and neurological system. Explain to the examiner what you are doing as you proceed and present your differential diagnosis.

NOTE

In the OSCE setting you will probably be expected to examine an adolescent teenager. However, it may be appropriate, particularly in the case of a young child, to ask a few questions of the parent regarding development and make general observations of the child at play before commencing your examination.

EXAMINATION

1 2 3

☐☐☐ **Introduction**   Introduce yourself. Establish rapport. Ascertain the patient's name and age. If an adult is present, confirm their relationship to the child.

Explain   Explain the purpose of the examination and obtain consent from the parent to expose and examine the child. Check that the child is comfortable.

Exposure   Position and expose the child's arms and legs adequately and appropriately.

EXAMINING GAIT

☐☐☐ **General**   Observe the child's limbs. Look for any wasting, fasciculation or hypertrophy.

☐☐☐ **Sitting**   Observe the child while they are sitting. Look for any postural abnormality or instability.

☐☐☐ **Rising**   Ask the child to stand up. Look specifically for Gower's sign whereby the child tries to elevate himself using his arms and hands to 'climb up' his body from squatting as a result of weak hip and thigh muscles (Duchenne muscular dystrophy).

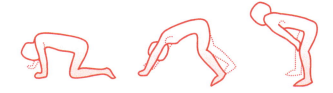

Gower's Sign

When the child is asked to stand up from the floor, the child attempts to elevate himself by holding onto and pushing off his thighs (limb girdle weakness – DMD).

☐☐☐ **Walking** — Ask the child to walk to the end of the room, turn round and return. Observe each stage of their gait including the start, rate, type of gait, arm swinging and how they turn around.

Observing the Child's Gait

Wide base/ataxic	Cerebellar disease
Hemiplegic	Stroke, infection, trauma, tumour, hemiplegic cerebral palsy
Spastic diplegic	(*Little's disease*) Spastic cerebral palsy
Painful/antalgic	Causes of pain: arthritis, sepsis, trauma
Limp and lurch	Unilateral hip dislocation
Waddling gait	Bilateral hip dislocation, muscular dystrophy (DMD)

ASSESSING NEUROLOGICAL FUNCTION

☐☐☐ **Tone** — Assess tone in the arms by asking the child to relax their arms by making them go 'floppy'. Gently test tone by flexing and extending the wrists and elbows while supinating and pronating the forearm. Assess tone in the legs by asking the child to relax their legs while you gently roll them back and forth with your hands.

☐☐☐ **Power** — Carry out a formal assessment of power if (as is likely) the child is old enough to follow your instructions. Each muscle should be tested in isolation. Compare both sides. For younger children it may be sufficient to assess them playing, for example, throwing or kicking a ball or picking up a toy from the floor.

Upper Limbs — Ensure that the child is sat upright before the examination.

Instructions to Assess Power in the Upper Limb

Shoulder abduction	'Raise your elbows like wings; don't let me push them down'
Elbow flexion	'Bring your arms up like a boxer; pull me towards you'
Elbow extension	'Push me away'
Long wrist extensors	'Make a fist with your hand and bend your wrist back; don't let me push it back down'
Finger extension	'Straighten your fingers and stop me from bending them when I push down'
Finger flexion	'Grab my fingers and squeeze them as hard as possible'
Finger abduction	'Spread your fingers wide apart and don't let me push them together'
Thumb abduction	'Raise your thumb to the ceiling and don't let me push it down'

Lower Limbs — Ensure that the child is lying flat when examining his lower limbs. Note that, if the child is very young, it is easier to observe their movements during physical activity and watch closely the relevant use of muscles against gravity.

Instructions to Assess Power in the Lower Limb

Hip flexion	Place hands on thigh. 'Push up against my hand'
Hip extension	Place hands under thigh. 'Push down against my hand'
Knee flexion	Bend child's knee and place a hand behind heel. 'Bring your heel to your bottom'
Knee extensors	Bend child's knee. 'Kick me away'
Ankle dorsiflexion	Hold child's medial and lateral malleoli with one hand. Place ulnar part of the other hand against the dorsal aspect of the foot. 'Push against my hand'
Ankle plantarflexion	Place ulnar part of hand against the plantar aspect of the foot. 'Push down against my hand'
Big toe extension	Place finger against the big toe. 'Push your toe against my finger'

☐ ☐ ☐ **Reflexes**   Use a tendon hammer to elicit reflexes in the arms (biceps, supinator and triceps) and legs (knee and ankle). Exaggerated reflexes are suggestive of an upper motor neurone lesion. Reduced reflexes are indicative of lower motor neurone lesion. Indicate that you would not try and elicit a plantar response as the Babinski test is not reliable in children.

Common Nerve Roots

MNEMONIC: NERVE ROOTS ASCEND FROM 1–8

Ankle S1, 2
Knee L3, 4
Supinator C5, 6
Biceps C5, 6
Triceps C7, 8

☐ ☐ ☐ **Coordination**   Test coordination in the upper and lower limbs. As with testing muscle power, a formal assessment is appropriate for children who can follow instructions effectively. Otherwise assess the child's coordination by asking the child to hop on one leg (lower limb) or to carry out a simple task like building blocks (upper limb).

Upper Limbs   Test finger-nose coordination by asking the child to move their index finger between your finger and their nose as fast as possible. Observe for past pointing and intention tremor. Test for dysdiadochokinesia by asking the child to clap their hand against their thigh alternating between dorsal and palmar surfaces (demonstrate this to the child).

Lower Limbs   Direct the child to move the heel of one foot and place it on the knee of the other leg. Next, ask them to run their heel down their shin and repeat the cycle again. Repeat the test on the other leg.

Sensation   A formal assessment of sensation is not usually required in an OSCE setting. However, do offer to perform a full sensory assessment.

☐☐☐ **Cranial Nerves**   A formal assessment of cranial nerve function is not usually required and is quite difficult to perform on an infant or toddler. Indicate to the examiner that you would like to carry out a full cranial nerve examination.

Assessing Cranial Nerves in an Infant or Child

I	Smell	Can be difficult to assess in a young child (try mint or vinegar)
II	Acuity, pupils	Can the child see? Perform visual test appropriate for age. Check direct and consensual light reflex as well as peripheral vision
III,IV,VI	Eye movements	Have the child follow your torch. Form an 'H' sign and observe the eye movements and ability to track your movements succinctly. Look for nystagmus
V	Sensation	Apply light touch to the child's face. Note a rooting reflex in a baby
VII	Facial muscles	Observe the child crying. Is there any facial asymmetry? Does the child close both eyes?
VIII	Hearing	Check the red book for formal hearing tests at birth. Consider distraction tests (infant) or audiometry tests
IX,X	Swallowing	Observe swallowing of water or bottle of milk
XI	Trapezius	Observe neck movements or ask child to shrug shoulders
XII	Tongue	Observe tongue movements or ask child to move protruded tongue from side to side

Request   State that you would request investigations as appropriate (imaging, nerve conduction, etc.) in order to confirm and support your diagnosis.

☐☐☐ **Summarise**   Check with the patient and deliver an appropriate summary.

EXAMINER'S EVALUATION

1 2 3 4 5
☐☐☐☐☐ Assessment of neurological system
☐☐☐☐☐ Role player's score
Total mark out of 23

DIFFERENTIAL DIAGNOSIS

Diagnosis	Symptoms	Management
Duchenne muscular dystrophy (DMD)	X-linked muscular dystrophy, 1 in 3000 male births. Mutation in dystrophin gene. Presents < 6 years old with proximal, symmetrical muscle weakness. Delayed walking, waddling gait, frequent falls and difficulty with stairs. Classic features: pseudohypertrophy of the calves, Gower's sign and muscle wasting.	CPK levels usually very high Genetic testing can be useful Echocardiogram and lung function testing annually. Supportive treatment and steroids are the mainstay of treatment. Most require wheelchair by 12. Average life expectancy is now between 25 and 30.
Becker's muscular dystrophy	Is the less severe form – rarely presents in childhood	As above – life expectancy near normal.
Cerebral palsy	Persistent, non-progressive motor syndromes affecting children < 3. Usually in utero cause. Prevalence is approximately 1 in 1000 live births. May be: spastic (70% of cases), choreoathetoid (dyskinetic) (10%) and ataxic (10%) or mixed (10%). Risk of CP include premature birth and low birth weight. Causes; prenatal cerebral malformation (60% of cases), injury during or after birth, infections, brain hypoxia and metabolic abnormalities. Typically non-progressive. Infant shows early hand preference (within 1 year), is stiff on handling and has late milestones. Symptoms include spastic tone, unsteady gait, involuntary movements, abnormal posture (adducted shoulder, flexed elbow and wrist with clenched hand), impaired coordination and abnormal tendon reflexes. In patients who are able to walk, a scissor gait and walking on toes are common. Associated features: occasionally severe learning difficulties, visual and hearing impairment, speech disorders, behavioural disorders and epilepsy.	There is no cure for CP and management is primarily based around improving the patient's quality of life and reducing symptoms through the use of physiotherapy, occupational and speech therapy. Associated conditions (e.g. epilepsy) are managed as necessary.

Diagnosis	Symptoms	Management
Myotonic dystrophy	Autosomal dominant inherited, chronic and progressive form of muscular dystrophy. Rare, 5 per 100 000. Usually appears between the ages of 15 and 40. Presenting features often include muscle weakness, stiffness and fatigue. Other features and associations include frontal balding, myopathic facies ('fish face'), sternocleidomastoid wasting (causing a 'swan neck' appearance), cataract formation, heart conduction defects and hypogonadism. Characteristically, sufferers have distal muscle weakness and wasting, and are unable to release their hands after grasping an object. Diverse cognitive problems may also be present.	Supportive management only.

3.9   PAEDIATRICS: INFANT AND CHILD BASIC LIFE SUPPORT

INSTRUCTIONS

You are leaving your busy paediatric outpatient clinic when you see a collapsed child in the waiting area. Nobody else is available for help. Assess the situation and commence resuscitation. (2015 Paediatric BLS guideline)

PROCEDURE

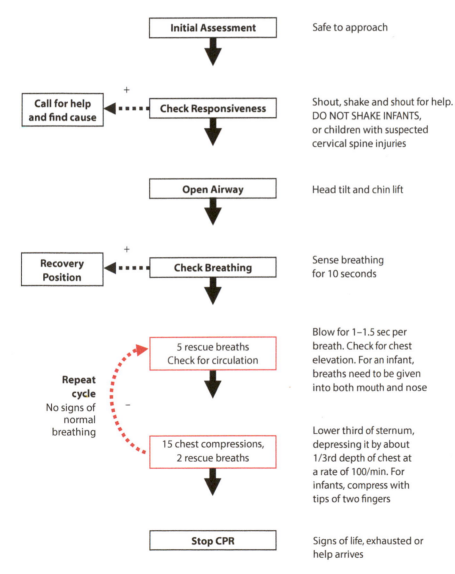

Initial Assessment → Safe to approach

Check Responsiveness → (+) **Call for help and find cause**
Shout, shake and shout for help. DO NOT SHAKE INFANTS, or children with suspected cervical spine injuries

Open Airway → Head tilt and chin lift

Check Breathing → (+) **Recovery Position**
Sense breathing for 10 seconds

5 rescue breaths / Check for circulation → Blow for 1–1.5 sec per breath. Check for chest elevation. For an infant, breaths need to be given into both mouth and nose

Repeat cycle No signs of normal breathing (–)

15 chest compressions, 2 rescue breaths → Lower third of sternum, depressing it by about 1/3rd depth of chest at a rate of 100/min. For infants, compress with tips of two fingers

Stop CPR → Signs of life, exhausted or help arrives

*Assessment Mnemonic – SSSS

1 2 3

☐☐☐ **Safe**　Ensure your own safety by confirming that it is safe to approach the patient. Check there is no immediate danger from the surroundings such as electricity, gas or chemical spillage.

☐☐☐ **Shout**　Check the responsiveness of the child by shouting, 'Are you all right?'

☐☐☐ **Stimulate**　Gently shake their shoulders or rub their sternum to see if there is a physical response. Do not shake if the casualty is an infant (1 year old or less), or a child with a suspected cervical spine injury.

☐☐☐ **Shout for Help**　If there is no response from the patient, shout for help.

　　　Responsive　If the patient is responsive (replies or moves), leave them in the position you found them, ensuring that the surrounding environment poses no danger. Try to establish the cause of the patient's current state and try to obtain assistance. Reassess the patient regularly in case of deterioration.

*Airway

☐☐☐ **Open Airway**　The patient should initially be left in the position they were found in. Open the airway by gently tilting the head back and lifting the chin. If you suspect a cervical spine injury then open the airway by jaw thrust only. The jaw thrust method may also be used if you encounter difficulty in opening the airway using the head-tilt, chin-lift method.

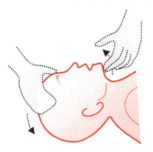

Airway Management
Open the patient's airway by placing your hand on his forehead and tilting the head backwards. Lift the chin by using your fingertips beneath it. In a suspected cervical spine injury, perform a jaw thrust only.

If you suspect that the neck has been injured, the airway should be opened using chin lift or jaw thrust alone. If in such a case the airway does not open, then the head should be tilted in small stages until the airway is opened.

*Breathing

☐☐☐ **Sense**　Keeping the airway open, bring your ear to the victim's mouth and sense for signs of breathing. Look for chest movements, listen for breath sounds and feel for breathing against your cheeks for no more than 10 seconds.

　　　Breathing　If the victim is breathing, reposition them into the recovery position and check for signs of continued breathing. Send for help or, if alone, seek assistance.

Not Breathing   If the child is not breathing normally, rescue breaths and assessment of circulation with subsequent chest compressions should be commenced before calling for help. In children and infants, five initial breaths should be given. Agonal gasps are infrequent, noisy breaths and should not be assumed to be evidence of normal breathing. This occurs in the minutes immediately after a cardiac arrest and should be treated as abnormal breathing.

□ □ □ **Technique**   Administer five rescue breaths appropriate for the child's age, employing the correct technique if they are neither breathing nor have agonal gasps.

Child (> 1 Year)   Maintain the airway by ensuring that the head is tilted and chin is lifted.

Pinch the patient's nose and place your lips around the mouth forming a good seal. For each breath, blow steadily for 1 making sure each breath causes the chest to rise and fall.

Head tilt and chin lift must be maintained even when your mouth leaves the patient and you are watching for the chest to fall. If a face mask is available, apply it over the patient's mouth before providing rescue breaths. Give five breaths overall and reassess.

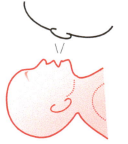

Assessing Breathing

Assess the patient's breathing by bringing your head to the patient's mouth and feeling for a breath against your cheek. Look for chest movements and listen for breath sounds for no more than 10 seconds. If in any doubt treat as if the patient's breathing is abnormal.

Infant (< 1 Year)   The head should be kept in a neutral position and chin lift should be applied.

Take a deep breath and form a tight seal over the mouth and nasal apertures of the infant.

Blow steadily for 1 second, making sure each breath causes the chest to rise and fall.

Take your mouth away and watch for his chest to fall as air comes out.

Repeat this five times overall and reassess.

Difficulty   Difficulty may be encountered if the airway is obstructed. In this case, look for any visible obstruction in the child's mouth but do not attempt a blind finger sweep. Check that the neck is not overextended. If head tilt and chin lift has not opened the airway, jaw thrust may be attempted.

Unsuccessful   Progress to chest compression if, after five attempts, you remain unsuccessful in achieving effective breaths.

*Circulation

☐☐☐ **Signs of Life**   Look for signs of movement, coughing or normal breathing. Agonal gasps do not count as signs of life.

☐☐☐ **Pulse**   Check the pulse for no more than 10 seconds.
In a child check the carotid pulse.
In an infant (< 1 year) palpate the brachial pulse.
Both can also supplement by checking the femoral pulse

Circulation   If there are signs of circulation present, continue rescue breaths until the child starts breathing on their own effectively. At this point, put the child in the recovery position and check for breathing regularly.

No Circulation   If there is no pulse, a slow pulse (< 60 bpm with poor perfusion) or if you are unsure about the pulse, chest compressions need to be started.

☐☐☐ **Technique**   Administer chest compressions appropriate for the child's age employing the correct technique if no signs of circulation are present.

All ages   In all children, compression of the upper abdomen needs to be avoided.
The xiphisternum should therefore be located and compressions should be performed one finger's breadth above this. Avoid the child's ribs, upper abdomen or base of the sternum.
Compress to 1/3 of the depth of the chest – 4 cm for an infant or 5 cm for a child.
A rate of 100–120 BPM should be used.
After 15 chest compressions give two breaths – continue at a ratio of 15:2.

Children   For small children older than 1 year, adequate compressions can be achieved using the heel of one hand only. Ensure that you are positioned vertically above the child's chest with your arm straightened, with your shoulder above your wrist and fingers lifted to avoid pressure over the ribs. Press down on the sternum, depressing the chest to about one-third of its depth, with the same duration taken for compression and release. If your hands and arms are too small or the child is too large for adequate compressions to be performed with one hand only, then both hands may be used with interlocked fingers. Take care not to apply pressure to the ribs.

Infants   For an infant, the tips of two fingers should be used rather than hands and arms, and ensure that the sternum is depressed by about one-third of the depth of the chest. If there are two or more rescuers, the 'encircling technique' can be employed. Place both thumbs flat, side by side, on the lower third of the sternum, with the tips pointing towards the infant's head. Encircle and support the infant's lower back with the rest of your fingers.

Two-finger Technique

Employ the two-finger technique on infants less than 1 year of age. Compress the chest by one-third of its depth with the tips of your index and middle finger over the sternum.

Hand-encircling Technique

Place both thumbs flat, side by side, on the lower third of the sternum, with the tips pointing towards the infant's head. Encircle and support the infant's lower back with the rest of your fingers. Depress the chest by one-third of the depth of the chest.

□□□ **Correct Ratio**   Two or more healthcare professionals should use a ratio of 15 compressions to two ventilations. If assistance is available, alternate chest compressors every two minutes to prevent exhaustion. Ensure the duration of the transitions is kept to a minimum.

□□□ **Call for Help**   One minute of CPR should be given before calling for help. Ask an individual to call the resuscitation team. If you are alone, leave the side of the victim and seek assistance by telephoning the emergency number. Dial 2222 (or equivalent).

'I am a foundation year House Officer in the paediatric outpatients' department. A child has collapsed in front of me and has no cardiac output. Please call the child resuscitation team immediately.'

□□□ **Repeat Cycle**   After completing 15 chest compressions, give the patient two effective rescue breaths. After providing two rescue breaths, continue with chest compressions. Maintain compressions at a rate of 100–120 per minute. If assistance is available, alternate chest compressors every 2 minutes to prevent exhaustion.

□□□ **Stop CPR**   Continue resuscitating the patient until help arrives, the victim shows signs of life (normal breathing, cough, movement or definite pulse of greater than 60 bpm) or you feel exhausted.

EXAMINER'S EVALUATION

1 2 3 4 5
□□□□□   Assessment of performance of paediatric BLS
           Total mark out of 24

3.10   PAEDIATRICS: EXPLAINING ASTHMA TO A CHILD

INSTRUCTIONS

You are a foundation year House Officer in general practice. Mr Durman and his 10-year-old son Thomas have attended clinic today for a follow-up to review the persistent night-time cough he has been experiencing for the past 2 months. Thomas has been diagnosed with asthma and Mr Durman is worried that it might affect his football. You will be marked on your communication skills and the information you provide.

HISTORY

1 2 3

☐ ☐ ☐   **Introduction**   Introduce yourself. Elicit the patient's name and age. Establish the adult's relationship to the child.

☐ ☐ ☐   **Ideas**   Explore parent and child's understanding of asthma.

'I understand that you have been complaining of a cough for the last 2 months and you have been told that you have asthma. Can you tell me what you understand by this?'

☐ ☐ ☐   **Concerns**   Elicit the parent and child's concerns about having asthma.
Expectations   Elicit patient's expectations of what they would like to achieve from the consultation today.

MEDICAL ADVICE

☐ ☐ ☐   **Explain**   Explain to the child what asthma is in a simple way, avoiding the use of jargon.

'When you breathe in, air passes from your mouth and into your lungs through a tube that looks like a big drinking straw. Your lungs are two big balloons filled up with lots of little tubes. In kids with asthma these tubes become smaller and tighter, making it hard for air to pass into your lungs. This is why you may cough, make a wheezy noise or find it hard to breathe.'

☐ ☐ ☐   **Treatment**   Establish the medication prescribed and explain the rationale behind the treatment of asthma.

'Your asthma medication makes it easier for you to breathe by opening up the tubes in the lungs. We normally use inhalers to treat asthma. These contain the medicine as a gas that you breathe into your lungs. There are two different types of inhalers, one blue and one brown. Normally we start you on the blue one, known as a reliever. This works by opening up the little tubes quickly and helps relieve your asthma straight away. The other type is the brown inhaler and is called a "preventer". This helps prevent your asthma from getting very bad and we normally give you this if you use your blue one too often.'

☐☐☐   **Monitoring**   Advise the patient when to attend the doctor for follow-up monitoring.

'It is important for your doctor to monitor your asthma regularly using a peak flow device, usually once or twice a year. However, there are particular occasions when you should visit your doctor; for example, if your asthma affects your school or sport activities; if it affects your sleep or if you find yourself using your inhaler three or more times a week. These situations may mean that your asthma is not well controlled and we may need to change your medication.'

☐☐☐   **Advice**   Offer appropriate advice to child and parent regarding cigarette-smoke exposure at home, regular dusting and cleaning (anti-mite cover for mattresses and pillows) and avoid keeping any pets in the bedroom.

Precipitating Factors for an Acute Asthma Attack

MNEMONIC: 'DIPLOMAT'

Drugs (aspirin, NSAIDs, beta blockers)
Infections (URTI, LRTI)
Pollutants
Laughter (emotion)
Oesophageal reflux (nocturnal asthma)
Mites
Activity and exercise
Temperature (cold)

☐☐☐   **Reassurance**   Reassure any parental concerns about asthma.

'Asthma is very common and is something you may have to live with for the rest of your life. If we took three children suffering with asthma, one child will ultimately grow out of it, the other may improve during their teen years only for the asthma to return in adulthood, and the last one will continue to be asthmatic. Even if you were to suffer with asthma for the rest of your life, you should be able to maintain a normal lifestyle. I understand that you have particular concerns about your son participating competitively in football tournaments. However, I would like to reassure you that there are a number of famous sport personalities who suffer with asthma, such as Paula Radcliffe and Paul Scholes, who continue to lead successful and fruitful lives.'

CLOSING

☐☐☐	**Understanding**	Confirm that the patient has understood what you have explained to them.
☐☐☐	**Questions**	Respond appropriately to the patient's questions.
	Leaflet	Offer to give them more information in the form of a handout. Advise that the leaflet contains much of the information you have mentioned.
☐☐☐	**Follow-up**	Offer the child and parent a follow-up appointment.

COMMUNICATION SKILLS

☐☐☐	**Rapport**	Maintain rapport and engage both the parent and the child throughout.
☐☐☐	**Fluency**	Speak fluently and do not use jargon.
☐☐☐	**Summarise**	Check with the patient and deliver an appropriate summary.

EXAMINER'S EVALUATION

1 2 3 4 5
☐☐☐☐☐ Overall assessment of explaining asthma to a child
☐☐☐☐☐ Role player's score
Total mark out of 28

3.11   PAEDIATRICS: EXPLAINING JAUNDICE

INSTRUCTIONS

You are a foundation year House Officer in general practice. Mrs Wilson gave birth to a baby boy 3 days ago. She has attended the practice and wishes to speak to a doctor as the baby has developed jaundice over the past day. It is otherwise healthy and doing well. Explain the possible causes of the baby's jaundice and deal with the mother's concerns appropriately. You will be assessed on your communication skills and on the information that you provide.

INTRODUCTION

1 2 3

☐☐☐ **Introduction**   Introduce yourself and establish rapport. Elicit the name of the mother and the age of the child and confirm their relationship.

☐☐☐ **Ideas**   Explore the mother's ideas of what may be causing her son's jaundice.

☐☐☐ **Concerns**   Elicit the mother's concern about her son's condition.

☐☐☐ **Expectations**   Elicit the mother's expectations from the consultation.

EXPLAINING JAUNDICE

☐☐☐ **Jaundice**   Explain what jaundice is, its causes and its significance in newborn babies.

'The yellow tinge that you have noticed in your child's skin and eyes is called jaundice. It occurs in about half of newborn babies. This form of jaundice is called physiological jaundice and is quite safe. It usually appears 2–3 days after birth, peaking after 5 days before gradually resolving within a couple of weeks without the need for treatment.'

'When the baby is in the womb it needs a higher number of red blood cells to carry oxygen around the body. Once it is born it can breathe oxygen on its own and so does not need as many red blood cells. These cells eventually get broken down by the body. When they get broken down a yellow substance called bilirubin is released. Usually this is carried to the liver. Sometimes in newborn babies the liver is not fully developed and so cannot get rid of this excess bilirubin which builds up and causes the yellowish appearance of the skin and sometimes in the whites of the eyes (sclera).'

☐☐☐ **Prolonged**   Explain to the patient what prolonged jaundice is.

'Jaundice can sometimes be prolonged for more than 2–3 weeks and this can occur if the baby has an infection. Occasionally, breast milk jaundice can occur and this is perfectly normal. The baby is healthy but produces low level of jaundice from the mother's milk. This type of jaundice usually clears up within 6 weeks. In such cases the mother may be asked to stop breast-feeding for a few days. Most of the other causes of jaundice are quite rare but may be serious. In such cases your baby may exhibit other symptoms, such as poor sucking or feeding and sleepiness.'

Diagnosis	Explain to the mother that their child is likely to be suffering from breast-milk jaundice.

EXPLAINING TREATMENT

☐☐☐ **Feeding** Explain that the mother should continue on with normal feeding.

'Since this form of jaundice is harmless to the baby, we advise you to continue breast-feeding or bottle feeding the baby.'

☐☐☐ **Blood Test** Explain when blood tests may be required.

'If the baby is unwell or not feeding, and if the jaundice does not improve within 2 weeks or begins to spread to include the arms or legs, or if the baby has pale stools and dark urine, you will need to bring him back to the GP. A blood test may be required to check the level of bilirubin in the blood.'

☐☐☐ **Treatment** Explain when phototherapy or exchange transfusion may be required.

'If the bilirubin level is found to be above a certain level (related to the child's age) the baby may require treatment. The main treatment of choice is known as phototherapy. This involves the baby lying naked with eyes covered, under a special ultraviolet lamp. The lamp produces a special light that converts the harmful pigment into a harmless form that is later excreted by the baby. On rare occasions where the bilirubin levels are very high an exchange transfusion may be required. This is where we need to take out some of the baby's blood containing the pigment and replace it with donor blood.'

☐☐☐ **Other Causes** Explain that there are other causes of jaundice in the newborn, and that treatment involves treating the cause.

'Other causes of jaundice in the newborn do exist but they are quite rare. They include infections, incompatibility between the baby's and mother's blood, metabolic abnormalities and liver disease or infection. I would like to reiterate that these causes are rare. If the jaundice is found to be due to such a cause, then treatment may involve medication or, in some cases, surgery.'

☐☐☐ **Complications** Explain that untreated persistent jaundice is potentially dangerous and should be treated.

'It is important to treat jaundice that is not mild and self-limiting, as in severe jaundice high levels of bilirubin can build up in the brain. If this is untreated, it can lead to brain damage and even death. I know that this sounds alarming but it is important to know that these complications (kernicterus) can be avoided if the jaundice is treated.'

Warning Signs   Explain to the mother that she should contact the GP or bring the baby in if the baby becomes ill or if the jaundice does not resolve.

'Please do not hesitate to bring your child in if he develops a fever, is not passing urine normally, or appears to be unwell, or if the jaundice does not resolve within 2 weeks.'

□□□   **Acknowledge**   Acknowledge and address the mother's concerns and reassure her.

'I appreciate your concerns and understand that there is a lot of information to take in. However, I would like to reassure you again that jaundice is quite common in babies, and as your child is otherwise doing well I suggest that you keep an eye on him for the next two weeks. If you have any concerns during that time please do not hesitate to call again as we are here to help.'

CLOSING

□□□   **Understanding**   Confirm that the patient has understood what you have explained to them.

□□□   **Questions**   Respond appropriately to the patient's questions.

Leaflet   Offer to give them more information in the form of a handout. Advise that the leaflet contains much of the information you have mentioned.

□□□   **Follow-up**   Offer the child and parent a follow-up appointment.

COMMUNICATION SKILLS

□□□   **Rapport**   Maintain rapport and engage both parent and child throughout.
□□□   **Fluency**   Speak fluently and do not use jargon.
□□□   **Summarise**   Check with the patient and deliver an appropriate summary.

EXAMINER'S EVALUATION

1 2 3 4 5
□□□□□   Assessment of explaining jaundice
□□□□□   Role player's score
         Total mark out of 30

DIFFERENTIAL DIAGNOSIS

Physiological

Physiological jaundice occurs in up to 50% of all infants. It reflects a temporary inadequacy of the immature liver in breaking down the erythrocytes following birth. Characteristically, jaundice is absent in the first 24 hours of life and often appears in the second or third day after birth. It occurs in a well child with serum bilirubin levels never reaching treatment levels. The condition completely resolves within 2 weeks of birth.

Prolonged Jaundice

Prolonged jaundice is considered to be jaundice lasting more than 14 days in full-term babies or more than 21 days in pre-term babies. Causes include physiological jaundice that has not resolved, breast milk, infection, hepatitis (neonatal), endocrine disease (hypothyroidism, hypopituitarism), choledochal cysts and an abnormal biliary tract (biliary atresia).

Early Neonatal Jaundice

Jaundice that is apparent in the first 24 hours of life is never physiological and is suggestive of haemolysis. Causes include haemolytic disease (ABO incompatibility, rhesus isoimmunisation), congenital infection (**mnemonic**: **TORCH** – **TO**xoplasmosis, **R**ubella, **C**MV, **H**erpes), haemolysis secondary to haematoma, Crigler–Najjar Syndrome, Dubin–Johnson Syndrome, Gilbert's Syndrome, transient familial hyperbilirubinaemia and maternal autoimmune haemolytic anaemia.

Conjugated Neonatal Jaundice

Conjugated neonatal jaundice occurs if conjugated bilirubin levels are more than 10% of total bilirubin or greater than 20µmol/L. It is always pathological. Causes include infection, sepsis, parenteral nutrition, cystic fibrosis, alpha-1 antitrypsin deficiency and endocrine and metabolic disease.

Kernicterus

The term 'kernicterus' is from the Greek words *kern* and *icterus* and literally means 'yellow kern' (deep nuclei). This refers to the high serum levels of unconjugated bilirubin that enter the nervous system and are deposited in the kern (basal ganglia, hippocampus, geniculate bodies and cranial nerve nuclei). Only unconjugated bilirubin can cross the blood-brain barrier. This rare condition may result in death or severe brain damage. It is often secondary to haemolytic diseases of the newborn such as rhesus isoimmunisation and G6PD deficiency.

3.12   PAEDIATRICS: EXPLAINING IMMUNISATIONS

INSTRUCTIONS

You are a foundation year House Officer in general practice. Mrs Wakefield has come into the practice with her newborn baby boy. She is aware that her son will require a programme of vaccinations, but does not know anything about them or when they are due. Advise Mrs Wakefield appropriately. You will be assessed on your communication skills and on the information that you provide.

INTRODUCTION

1 2 3

☐☐☐ **Introduction**   Introduce yourself. Elicit the patient's name, age and occupation. Establish rapport.

☐☐☐ **Ideas**   Explore the mother's understanding of immunisations.

'Congratulations on the birth of your new baby. I understand that you have come in today to discuss your child's immunisations, which are now due. Can you tell me what you already know about immunisations?'

☐☐☐ **Concerns**   Elicit her concerns and explore them appropriately.

'Is there anything in particular that worries you about immunisations?'

Expectations   Elicit the mother's expectations of what she would like to achieve from the consultation today.

MEDICAL ADVICE

☐☐☐ **Immunisation**   Briefly explain what immunisations are and how vaccines work.

'Immunisations give our body the ability to fight certain diseases if we come into contact with them. This is done by injecting a vaccine, which contains a tiny part of a bacterium, virus or their products. This small substance is not enough to make you unwell. However, it does allow the body to prepare a defence response and recognise the disease. If the child were to come in contact with the real disease, the immune system would be prepared to fight against the infection by using small proteins called antibodies and thereby protect the child.'

☐☐☐ **Programme**   Explain the diseases that the childhood immunisation programme would protect against.

Childhood Immunisation Programme (UK)

List of immunisations that are offered to children

Diphtheria	Whooping cough (pertussis)
Tetanus	Measles
Mumps	Rubella (German measles)
Meningitis C as infant*	Pneumococcal infection
Meningitis ACWY at 14 years	Haemophilus influenzae type B (Hib)

2015: Meningitis B has been added to infant regime

Polio

Influenza from 2 to 6 years old

HPV from 12 to 14 years for girls

☐ ☐ ☐ **Timing** Explain the ages at which the vaccines should be given and the importance of giving them at the right time.

'The vaccination programme is started when the child is still young. This is because the diseases can be very serious in childhood. It is therefore necessary to provide them with protection as early as possible.

'The first immunisations are performed when the baby is aged 2 months. Further doses are given at the ages of 3 months and 4 months. Additional immunisations are given around the ages of 12 months and 13 months, as well as at preschool (3.5–5 years) and finally, during the teens. We also recommend annual flu vaccination for children from two to six years old.'

☐ ☐ ☐ **Multiple Doses** Explain why multiple doses of certain vaccines are required.

'For adequate protection, your child's immune system needs to be fully prepared against the specific diseases that we are trying to protect against. This is why for most immunisations more than one dose is needed. For long-term protection, booster doses are given later on in life.'

☐ ☐ ☐ **Effectiveness** Explain the effectiveness of the immunisation programme.

'The UK immunisation programme has been very successful at reducing the incidence of infectious diseases in children. Because of the immunisation programme, some serious diseases such as diphtheria have almost disappeared from this country. Even though these diseases are now uncommon in the UK, they cause serious illness and death in millions of children under the age of five around the world. In most cases these deaths can be prevented by immunisation. Nowadays, there is a lot of travelling to and from the UK and there is a risk that the disease may be brought into the UK. The vaccines protect against this risk.'

☐ ☐ ☐ **Side Effects** Explain that the vaccination may cause mild side effects in some children.

'The vaccines may produce mild side effects. In most cases, the child may become a little irritable and feel unwell. Some redness and swelling may appear at the site of the injection. Some babies may also develop a fever. If your child does develop a fever, you may consider giving them paracetamol to reduce it.'

ADDRESS CONCERNS

☐☐☐ **Concerns**   Address the mother's concerns appropriately including the
                          number of vaccines, allergies and drug safety issues.

       Overloading   Explain to the mother that having multiple vaccines does not
                          overload the child's immune system.

'There are hundreds of thousands of young children who have successfully gone through the UK childhood immunisation programme without any problems. Vaccines are designed to make the baby's immune system stronger, and there is no evidence that multiple vaccines overload the immune system. I would like to point out that the risk of serious harm resulting because of non-immunisation is far greater than any potential risk from having multiple vaccines.'

       Allergies   Explain that common allergies are not a contraindication to
                         vaccines. Mention that in only rare circumstances are vaccines
                         withheld.

No Obligation   Mention that although it is highly recommended, in the UK,
                         parents can decide not to have their child immunised. Reiterate
                         that immunisation is the best choice as it protects against serious
                         and potentially fatal diseases.

CLOSING

☐☐☐ **Understanding**   Confirm that the patient has understood what you have
                         explained to them.

☐☐☐ **Questions**   Respond appropriately to the patient's questions.
       Leaflet   Offer to give them more information in the form of a handout.
                         Advise that the leaflet contains much of the information you
                         have mentioned.

☐☐☐ **Follow-up**   State that appointments and an immunisation schedule will be
                         made for the child and can be found in their red book. Arrange a
                         follow-up, if appropriate.

COMMUNICATION SKILLS

☐☐☐ **Rapport**   Maintain rapport and engage both parent and child throughout.
☐☐☐ **Fluency**   Speak fluently and do not use jargon.
☐☐☐ **Summarise**   Check with the patient and deliver an appropriate summary.

EXAMINER'S EVALUATION

1 2 3 4 5
☐ ☐ ☐ ☐ ☐   Overall assessment of explaining immunisation
☐ ☐ ☐ ☐ ☐   Role player's score
Total mark out of 30

CHILDHOOD INFECTIONS

Infection	Organism	Spread	Incubation period	Symptoms	Vaccine
Diphtheria	Corynebacterium diphtheriae	Spread by direct physical contact or breathing in the vapourised secretions of infected individuals	2–5d	Upper respiratory tract illness. Initial sore throat and generalised symptoms such as fever and rigors. These can worsen and cause severe breathing difficulties associated with lymphadenopathy and acute epiglottitis. In serious cases it can cause cardiomyopathy, peripheral neuropathy and even death.	DTaP 2,3,4 months and 3 years Td/IPV at 14 years
Pertussis (whooping cough)	Bordetella pertussis	Airborne via droplet discharges	2d	Catarrhal stage: cough, sneezing and a runny nose > paroxysmal stage: characteristic cough with fits of coughing sometimes associated with vomiting and choking. May last 10 weeks. Complications – pulmonary hypertension and encephalitis.	DTaP 2,3,4 months and 3 years
Tetanus	Clostridium tetani	Wound contamination and neurotoxin release	3–21d	Classic – lockjaw followed by spasms in the rest of the body and breathing difficulties. Seizures. 10% mortality.	DTaP 2,3,4 months and 3 years Td/IPV at 14 years
Polio	Poliovirus	Faeco-oral route	2–20d	Asymptomatic – initial flu-like illness. 3% have CNS involvement – non-paralytic aseptic meningitis or paralytic poliomyelitis – which can be spinal, bulbospinal or bulbar. Complications: paralysis, cardiac arrest, respiratory failure and death. Last UK case 1984.	DTaP 2,3,4 months and 3 years Td/IPV at 14 years
Hib (Haemophilus influenzae type B)	Haemophilus influenzae (bacterium)	Encapsulated organism – spread via airdrops.	< 5d	Septicaemia, pneumonia and meninigitis. Can be fatal. Particular risk in asplenic patients, e.g. sickle cell.	Hib 2,3,4 and 12 months
Pneumococcus	Streptococcus pneumoniae	Mainly droplet spread – common throat carriage	< 5d	Pneumonia, otitis media and meningitis. More common in young children and the elderly.	PCV 2,4 and 12 months

Infection	Organism	Spread	Incubation period	Symptoms	Vaccine
Measles	Paramyxovirus	Respiratory spread by airborne droplets	7–14d	Initial prodrome of malaise, fever and three Cs: cough, coryza and conjunctivitis. Koplik spots appear on the buccal and lingual mucosa (opposite the lower 1st and 2nd molars). 2–3d later> maculopapular rash. Infectious 1/52 later. Usually self-limiting – complications include pneumonitis, encephalitis and subacute sclerosing pan encephalitis – very rare but neurologically debilitating delayed onset illness (see below)	MMR 13 months, 3 years and top-up 14 years
Mumps	Paramyxovirus	Transmission is via airborne droplet spread	14–25d	30% of cases asymptomatic. Infectious 3d prior to 10d post illness. Initial symptoms: fever, general malaise, a sore throat, a dry mouth, myalgia, fatigue and headaches. Parotid inflammation can last for up to a week. Meningitis occurs in 15–20% of individuals with mumps, rarely serious. Orchitis is commoner in post-pubescent individuals. Treatment is supportive although complications require specific management.	MMR 13 months, 3 years and top-up 14 years
Rubella (German measles)	Togavirus	Airborne droplet transmission	14–21d	Usually mild in nature, with a general increase in severity of symptoms with age. Prodromal phase: general malaise, fever and headache. 2–3d: Pink macular rash starting on the face, spreading to the trunk and limbs and then slowly fading away. Associated with cervical lymph node enlargement, particularly of the sub-occipital and post-auricular nodes. Forchheimer's sign refers to discrete rose-coloured petechiae on the soft palate although this is not specific to rubella. Infectivity is greatest just prior to the onset of symptoms. Diagnosis: rubella IgM + characteristic rash. Treatment is supportive plus contact isolation, partciularly from pregnant women.	MMR 13 months, 3 years and top-up 14 years

Complications of Measles

MNEMONIC: 'MEASLES COMPLICATION'

Myocarditis
Encephalitis
Appendicitis
Subacute sclerosing panencephalitis
Laryngitis
Early death
Shits (diarrhoea)
Corneal ulcer
Otis media
Mesenteric lymphadenitis
Pneumonia (bronchiolitis, bronchitis, croup)

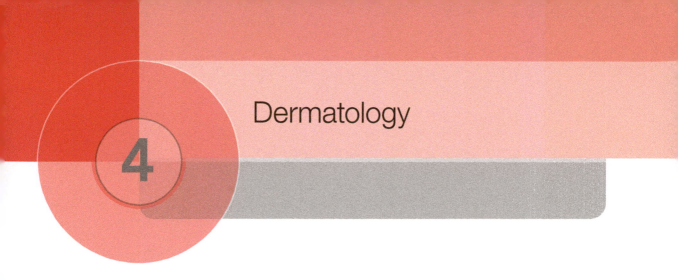

Dermatology

4.1   DERMATOLOGY: DERMATOLOGICAL HISTORY

INSTRUCTIONS

You are a foundation year House Officer in dermatology. You are asked to see Miss Catteo, a 30-year-old lifeguard, in the clinic. Take a full dermatology history, present your findings and give differential diagnoses to the examiner.

INTRODUCTION

☐☐☐ **Introduction**   Introduce yourself appropriately and establish rapport with the patient.

☐☐☐ **Name and Age**   Elicit the patient's name and age.

☐☐☐ **Occupation**   Enquire about the patient's occupation.

FOCUSED HISTORY

☐☐☐ **Skin Problem**   What seems to be the problem? Can you describe your skin problem? Where is it? When did it first start? Has it changed over time? Has it spread to other areas?

☐☐☐ **Exacerb./reliev.**   Does anything make it better or worse (cream, sunlight, heat, soaps)?

☐☐☐ **Assoc. Sympt.**   Are there any associated symptoms (itching, pain, exuding, blistering, bleeding)? Have you noticed any problems with your nails, joints, scalp or hair?

☐☐☐ **Medical History**   Have you had any similar episodes of this in the past? Have you had any other skin problems in the past? Do you have any allergies? Do you suffer from asthma, hayfever or eczema? Do you have any other medical conditions?

☐☐☐ **Family History**   Do you have a family history of any skin conditions such as psoriasis, eczema or skin cancers?

☐☐☐ **Drug History**   Have you tried any medication or creams for your skin problem? Do you use cosmetics or moisturising creams? Do you have any skin (nickel) or drug allergies?

Drug-Induced Skin Reactions

Exanthematous reactions	Allopurinol, furosemide, phenytoin
Fixed drug eruption	Tetracycline, ibuprofen, sulphonamide, barbiturates
Urticaria/angiooedema	Penicillin, codeine, aspirin, anti-epileptics
Psoriasiform eruptions	ACE inhibitors, beta blockers, tetracycline, lithium
Purpura	Aspirin, quinine, sulphonamides, atropine, penicillin
Vasculitis	Allopurinol, carbamazepine, NSAIDs, thiazides
Erythema multiforme	Co-trimoxazole, lamotrigine, macrolides
Photosensitivity	Amiodarone, thiazide, tetracyclines, sulphonylurea
Alopecia	Antidepressants, cimetidine, lithium, valproate, warfarin
Nail disorders	Chloramphenicol, chlorpromazine, phenytoin

☐☐☐ **Social History** Does your skin problem have any relationship to your work? What does your job actually involve you doing? Do you have any particular hobbies? Do you come into contact with animals? Do you travel extensively? Do you get a lot of sun exposure? Do you smoke or drink alcohol?

☐☐☐ **Idea** What do you think may be causing this skin problem? Are there any particular concerns?

☐☐☐ **Impact on Life** How has this problem affected your life?

COMMUNICATION SKILLS

☐☐☐ **Rapport** Establish and maintain rapport with the patient and demonstrate listening skills.

☐☐☐ **Response** React positively to and acknowledge the patient's emotions.

☐☐☐ **Fluency** Speak fluently and do not use jargon.

☐☐☐ **Summarise** Check with the patient and deliver an appropriate summary.

'This is Miss Catteo, a 30-year-old lifeguard, who presents with a history of a spot on her cheek that has slowly increased in size. She mentions that the lesion is getting redder, is ulcerative and has a shiny appearance. Although she was born in London, she spent most of her adult life in Australia where she worked as a life guard. She states that she spends a lot of time in the sun, but uses sunscreen regularly. There is no history of skin cancer in the family nor does she have any medical complaints (renal transplant, immunosuppression). She is extremely concerned that her skin problem is cancerous and may require an operation. In view of her history, I suspect that she may be suffering from a basal cell carcinoma (BCC). I would like to perform a biopsy to exclude other differentials such as actinic keratosis, Bowen's disease, squamous cell carcinoma and eczema.'

EXAMINER'S EVALUATION

1 2 3 4 5

☐☐☐☐☐ Overall assessment of dermatology history

☐☐☐☐☐ Role player's score

Total mark out of 29

DIFFERENTIAL DIAGNOSIS

Condition	Incidence	Symptoms
Acne vulgaris	> 85% – common in both male and females – peak age at 18 and around puberty	Characterised by papules, open and closed comedones (blackheads and whiteheads), pustules, nodules and scars in the sebaceous gland distribution such as the face, neck, back and chest. Abscesses and sinuses with scarring (conglobate acne) are seen only in the most severe presentations. Colonisation with propionibacterium acnes. Associated with PCOS, Cushing's, congenital adrenal hyperplasia drugs including steroids and androgens.
Pityriasis rosea	0.3–3% – common at GPs and dermatology centres	Presents as a pink and flaky oval-shaped herald patch between 2 and 5 cm in diameter. Several days later, smaller cluster patches develop over the trunk, upper arms and thighs in a triangular pattern, like a Christmas tree. A severe itch often precedes the rash.
Pityriasis (tinea) versicolor	Up to 50% in warm tropical countries e.g. Samoa	Benign fungal infection – Malassezia sp. presents with varying colours and shapes. It manifests as a macular rash of different pigmentation to the patient's skin, with well-defined margins. The lesions are often finely scaly, brownish pink in colour and oval or round on untanned skin. In darker skin, the lesions are more evident with a hypopigmented quality. However, each individual's lesions are evenly pigmented and lack any of the erythema or central clearing that is commonly seen in most fungal infections. Trunk > spread to the proximal limbs.

Image	Treatment
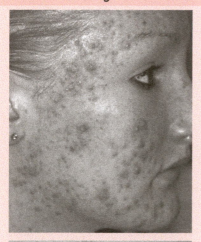	Escalating treatment based on severity and response. Simple hygiene measures. Topical agents – including salicylates, antibiotics and retinoids. Systemic treatment includes antibiotics, anti-androgen contraceptive pill e.g. cyproterone acetate or oral isotretinoin – patient must *not* be pregnant if oral retinoid is prescribed.
	Self-limiting.
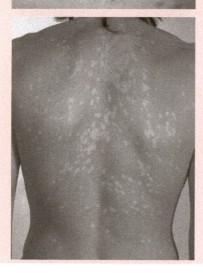	Topical antifungal for 2/52 and then oral antifungal for resistant cases.

Lichen planus	Affects men and women equally but is more common in middle-aged adults.	Resemblance tree moss hence the name. It presents as shiny itchy flat-topped (2–5 mm) polygonal lesions over flexor surfaces including the palm, soles, mucous membranes and genitalia. Violaceous (violet, bluish purple) colour. Oral lichen planus is the most common presentation and manifests as lacy streaks called Wickham's striae.
Pemphigus vulgaris	Middle-aged adult	Comprises a group of rare autoimmune disorders that cause blistering of the skin and mucous membranes due to antibodies directed at the basement membrane. Presents as sores in the mouth that make eating and chewing painful > widespread flaccid superficial bullae particularly affecting the scalp, chest, back and face. Blisters may burst to form crusted erosions.
Bullous pemphigoid	Affects people up to 65 years old	It presents as an urticarial reaction with significant pruritus that rapidly develops into large, tender, tense, dome-shaped bullae ranging from 1 to 6 cm affecting the flexor surfaces and trunk. It is characterised by periods of exacerbation and remission with episodes lasting 1–5 years. Future recurrences are often mild and less severe.
Basal cell carcinoma (BCC)	Elderly or middle-aged subjects – most common malignancy of the skin	Slow-growing, locally invasive, but rarely metastasizing, tumour that arises from a subset of the basal cells in the epidermis. The main cause of BCC is prolonged ultraviolet exposure such that these tumours are more common in fair-skinned people living near the equator. BCC is seen typically on the face (commonly around the nose, the inner canthus of the eyelids and the temples). Occasionally scalp, behind the ear and on the trunk. There are a number of clinical variants of BCC, the nodular type being by far the most common variety. This type of BCC usually presents as a nodule (pictured) with a pearly, rolled edge and telangiectatic vessels on the surface.

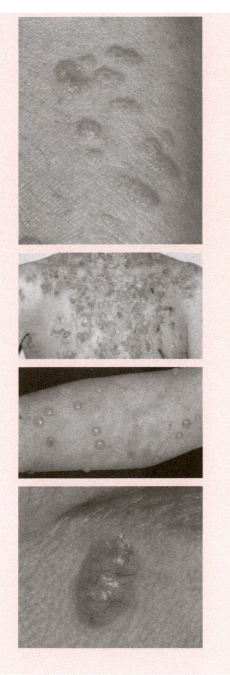

The condition is often self-limiting but steroids can be used to reduce the effects of inflammation.

Can range from mild disease requiring topical steroid to life-threatening disease requiring systemic steroids, immunosuppression and plasmaphoresis.

Again mild disease requires topical steroids – severe or resistant disease requires systemic immunosuppression and maintenance.

Local excision with a 2–4 mm margin is treatment of choice. Recurrence unlikely if completely resected. Mohs procedure for areas where easy margins not possible, e.g. nose.

Lichen Planus

Characteristics of Lichen Planus

MNEMONIC: '5 PS OF PLANUS'

Peripheral (palm, soles)
Polygonal (2–5 mm)
Plane (flat topped)
Pruritic in nature
Purple (violaceous)

4.2   DERMATOLOGY: DERMATOLOGICAL EXAMINATION

INSTRUCTIONS

You are a foundation year House Officer in dermatology. You are asked to see Mr Bowen, a 55-year-old man, in the clinic. Carry out a full dermatology examination. Present your findings and give a differential diagnosis to the examiner.

INTRODUCTION

1 2 3

□□□	**Introduction**	Introduce yourself appropriately and establish rapport with the patient.
□□□	**Name and Age**	Elicit the patient's name and age.
□□□	**Occupation**	Enquire about the patient's occupation.

EXAMINATION

	Consent	Explain the examination to the patient and obtain his consent.
□□□	**Prepare**	Ensure that there is adequate illumination (skin needs to be examined in good light – preferably natural). Adequately expose the patient (ideally the patient should be undressed to his undergarments). Ask the patient if there is any pain or tenderness before commencing your examination.

*Inspection

□□□	**Observe**	Observe the skin and determine what type of lesions there are, their site, distribution, size, shape and colour.

Inspection in Dermatological Examination

Site	Describe the exact position(s) of the skin lesion(s): Flexor/extensor surfaces, ventral/dorsal surfaces Proximal/distal to nearest bony landmark
Location	Face/trunk/limbs/buttocks/scalp/ears/neck/nape/axillae/groins/arms/forearms/ legs/thighs/palms/soles/knees/ankles/wrists/elbows/cubital fossae/popliteal fossae
Hands/feet	Palmar/dorsal surface of hands, plantar/dorsal surface of feet
Distribution	Single/multiple, unilateral/bilateral, symmetrical/asymmetrical
	Discrete/confluent/localised/grouped/generalised/scattered/diffuse
	Dermatomal/photo-distribution (sun-exposed areas)
Size	Measure exact dimensions using a ruler: small/large/varying sizes
Shape	Spherical/hemispherical
	Oval/circular/annular (ring-like)/nummular (coin-like)/discoid (disc-like)
	Irregular/polygonal (multisided)/monomorphic (one form)/polymorphic (varying)
	Linear/curvilinear/arcuate (curved), reticular (net-like)/serpiginous (serpent-like)

Colour	Flesh-coloured (normal skin colour)
	Hyper-pigmented (darker than normal)/hypopigmented (paler than normal)
	Erythematous (red)/violaceous (violet)/purpuric (purple)
	White/yellow/orange/pink/pearly/translucent/brown/black

*Palpation

☐ ☐ ☐ **Skin Lesion** — Gently palpate the skin to assess the type of lesion present. Consider wearing gloves if you are examining an erosion or ulceration.

Macule — Flat, non-palpable, circumscribed area of skin discolouration.

Common Differentials of a Macular Rash

Drug reaction	History of drugs (antibiotics, thiazide), fever, affects trunk and limbs
	Distribution morbilliform (measles-like), urticarial or erythema multiforme
Freckles	Facial, small, light brown macules, darken in sun, common in redheads
Pityriasis rosea	Adolescent, generalised eruption preceded by herald patch (large 2–5 cm oval lesion), lesions are oval, pink, scaly, itchy
Pity. versicolor	Fungal (*Pityrosporum orbiculare*), adolescents, hypopigmented patches in darker skin, affects trunk and proximal limbs
Vitiligo	Well-defined white macules, no melanocytes, hands, face (eyes and mouth)
Café au lait spots	Neurofibromatosis, oval-shaped creamy brown patches (pictured)

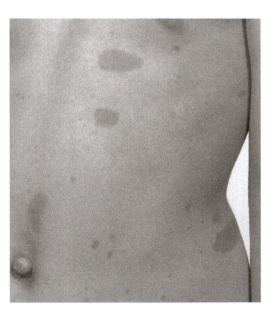

Fig. 4.1 Café au lait spots

Plaque — Solid, palpable, flat-topped, area of skin elevation > 5 mm diameter.

Common Differentials of Scales and Plaques

Psoriasis	Well-defined, erythematous coloured waxy disc-shaped plaques with silver scales, extensor surfaces and scalp, itchy
Eczema	History of asthma or hayfever, itchy, dry skin, excoriation, flexor surfaces
Fungal (tinea)	Affects trunk or limbs (corporis), groin (cruris), feet (pedis), scalp (capitis) Singular/multiple annular-shaped erythematous scaly plaques, defined margins, clear centrally. Alopecia if it affects the scalp

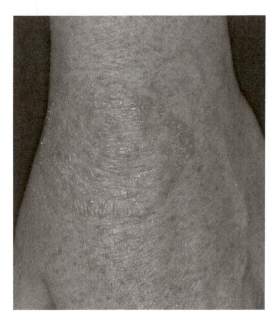

Fig. 4.2 Tinea corporis

Papule   Solid, raised, palpable skin lesion < 5 mm diameter.

Common Differentials of Papules

Acne vulgaris	Puberty, comedogenic areas (face, back, chest), greasy skin, blackheads and whiteheads, papules, pustules, cysts and scars
Scabies	Mite (*Sarcoptes scabiei*), intense itch, burrow (tortuous small ridge – 1 cm), affects fingers, wrists, nipples, does not occur above neck
Moll. contagiosum	Viral (pox virus), pearly pink, 1–3 mm diameter, umbilicated papules, contain cheesy material, itchy, grouped lesions on truck, face, neck
Guttate psoriasis	Adolescent, history of throat infection (beta haemolytic streptococcus), widespread raindrop-shaped pink papules over trunk or limbs
Lichen Planus	Itchy, shiny, polygonal, flat-topped (2–5 mm), white streaks (Wickham's striae), red papules turn violaceous, flexor surfaces, palm, soles, mucous membrane
Milia	Children, small white raised spots on face (upper cheeks and eyelids)
Urticaria	Superficial itchy pink swelling (wheals) with some papules, deep swelling (angiooedema) of tongue or lips, food (peanut) or drug (penicillin) reaction

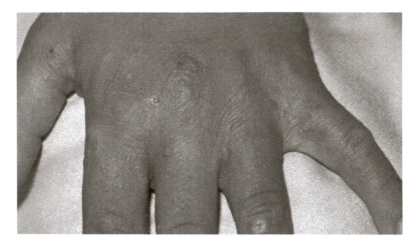

Fig. 4.3 Scabies rash

Nodule   Solid, raised, palpable skin lesion > 5 mm diameter.

Common Differentials of Nodules

Sebaceous cyst	Firm, smooth, oval-shaped, intradermal, visible punctum
Keloid scar	Proliferation of connective tissue, firm smooth nodules, history of trauma
Seborrhoeic wart	Papillary surface with keratin plug, defined margin, 'stuck on' appearance, pedunculated and protuberant, affects face, neck or trunk
Lipoma	Benign tumour of fat, soft masses, multiple, trunk, neck, upper extremities
Dermatofibroma	Firm nodule, commonly lower legs, history of trauma or insect bite
BCC	Pearly nodules, reddish colour, ulcer with rolled edge, sun-exposed areas
SCC	> 55 yrs, actinic keratosis progresses to ulcerate and crust, sun-exposed areas
Keratoacanthoma	Rapidly growing nodule, keratin plug or crater, sun-exposed areas

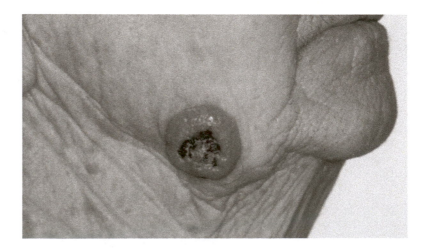

Fig. 4.4 Keratoacanthoma

| *Vesicle* | Fluid-filled (serous), raised, palpable skin lesion < 5 mm diameter. |
| *Bulla* | Fluid-filled (serous), raised, palpable skin lesion > 5 mm diameter. |

Common Differentials for Blisters (Vesicle and Bulla)

Insect bites	Depending on the insect, a blister, papules or urticarial wheal can occur
Herpes simplex	Itchy and tender clusters of tense vesicles with erythematous base, yellow crust formation, recurrent infections
Chickenpox	Prodromal illness (fever and pain), erythematous lesions develop into vesicles, pustules and dry crusts, crops of blisters affect trunk, face, limbs, scalp
Shingles (HZV)	Unilateral groups of vesicles in a dermatome with late scabs, very tender
Dermatitis herpetiformis	Coeliac disease, symmetrical, trunk and extensor surface, itchy vesicular rash
Pemphigus	Seen in the middle-aged, widespread flaccid superficial bullae, blisters and erosions, mucous membrane, Nikolsky sign
Pemphigoid	Seen in the elderly, urticarial reaction rapidly develops into tense bullae, flexor surfaces and trunk, recurrent and more common than pemphigus

| *Pustule* | Vesicle or bulla containing purulent fluid. |

Common Differentials of Pustules

Impetigo	*S. aureus*, thin-walled blisters rupture forming yellow crust lesions, contagious
Boil, carbuncle	*S. aureus* infection of hair follicle, hard tender red nodule, increase in size, pus
Pustular psoriasis	Unwell, fever, small yellow pustules on erythematous base, commonly over palmar and plantar aspects, rapid spread
Acne vulgaris	As described as above
Rosacea	Erythema, telangiectasia, pustules, papules and oedema, affects cheeks, nose and forehead, rhinophyma (bulbous appearance of nose)

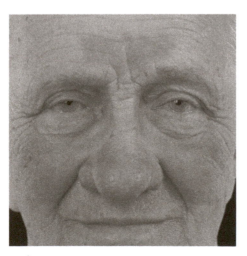

Fig. 4.5 Erythematous rosacea

	Erosion	Area of skin denuded by partial or complete loss of epidermis.
	Fissure	Slit in epidermis.
	Ulcer	Area of skin denuded by loss of epidermis and loss of underlying dermis.
	Wheal	Elevated area of cutaneous oedema with pale centre and pink rim.
	Petechia	Pinhead-sized macule of blood in skin that blanches on pressure.
	Purpura	Larger macule/papule of blood in skin that does not blanch on pressure.
	Ecchymosis	Larger extravasation of blood in skin (bruise).
	Telangiectasia	Visible dilatation of small cutaneous blood vessels.
☐☐☐	**Edge**	Describe the edge as well-circumscribed, ill-defined or irregular.
☐☐☐	**Surface**	Describe the surface of the skin lesion.

Palpation in a Dermatological Examination

Surface	Smooth/rough/hard/soft/xerotic (dry)/wet/exudative
	Excoriation (superficial abrasion due to scratching)
	Atrophic (thinning of skin)/indurated (hardening of skin)
	Scaly (flakes due to shedding of epidermal cells)/crusted (dried exudate)
	Maceration (softening/disintegration of skin following prolonged wetting)
	Lichenification (increased epidermal thickness with accentuated skin markings)
	Flat-topped/umbilicated (central depression)/acuminate (pointed, spire-like)
	Pedunculated (with a stalk)/sessile (without a stalk)/verrucous (warty)

☐☐☐	**2° Sites**	Look for associated features. In psoriasis, check for involvement of scalp, nails (pitting, onycholysis) and distal interphalangeal joints of the hands (arthropathy). In lichen planus, check for involvement of the oral mucosa (Wickham's striae), hair (scarring alopecia) and nails (nail dystrophy).

Common Causes of Hair, Sweat Gland Problems and Nail Changes

Alopecia	Hair loss can be diffuse or localised
Diffuse	Genetic, hypothyroidism, malnutrition, iron deficiency, drug-induced
Localised	Alopecia areata, tinea capitis (ringworm), SLE, trauma, secondary syphilis
Hirsutism	Excess hair in androgenic distribution. Idiopathic, drugs (phenytoin, corticosteroids), PCOS, menopause, Cushing's syndrome, ovarian cancer
Hypertrichosis	Excess hair in non-androgenic distribution (face and trunk)
	Drugs (phenytoin), malnutrition, anorexia nervosa, porphyria
Hyperhidrosis	Excess sweating. Physiological, menopause, malaria, thyrotoxicosis
Onycholysis	Separation of nail from nail bed. Psoriasis, fungal, thyrotoxicosis, trauma
Koilonychia	Spoon-shaped nails. Iron deficiency anaemia, lichen planus
Pitting	Psoriasis, eczema, lichen planus

☐☐☐	**Lymph Nodes**	In suspected skin malignancy, examine the regional lymph nodes for lymphadenopathy. Check as well for hepatomegaly and splenomegaly.

☐☐☐   **Summarise**   Summarise your findings to the examiner.

'This is Mr Bowen, a 55-year-old builder, who has been suffering from a red/silver scaly lesion on both extensor surfaces of his elbows. The right lesion measures 7 cm by 4 cm while the left measures 4 cm by 3 cm. Both lesions are oval in shape and are scaly in appearance. He also complains of nail changes. On examination, he was found to have widespread pitting and onycholysis. On direct questioning, he mentioned that the lesions were initially small but got worse when he started taking beta blockers for his angina. In view of the examination, I suspect Mr Frank suffers from psoriasis, however, I would like to rule out atopic dermatitis and eczema.'

EXAMINER'S EVALUATION

1 2 3 4 5

☐☐☐☐☐   Overall assessment of dermatology examination
☐☐☐☐☐   Role player's score
                Total mark out of 27

DIFFERENTIAL DIAGNOSIS

Psoriasis

Psoriasis is a chronic skin condition characterised by inflamed, red, raised areas that develop as silvery scales on the scalp, elbows, knees and lower back. Around 2% of the population have psoriasis. Alcohol, beta blockers, lithium, NSAIDs and antimalarials can exacerbate the condition. The most common form is called discoid or plaque psoriasis. Symptoms include salmon-coloured plaques with silver-white scales on the extensor surfaces as well as the scalp that are often itchy in nature. Other types include guttate and pustular psoriasis. Guttate psoriasis affects mostly teenagers and presents with multiple drop-like lesions that occur after a streptococcal throat infection. Pustular psoriasis presents with small pustules (pus-containing blisters) that can appear all over the body or on just the palms, soles and other small areas. Psoriasis can also involve the nails (in 50% of cases) as well as the joints (7%). Nail features include pitting, ridging, onycholysis (separation of distal nail from the nail bed) and hyperkeratosis (build up of keratin below the nail bed).

Eczema

Eczema is a term used for many types of skin inflammation (dermatitis) including atopic (the commonest), contact, allergic, seborrhoeic and stasis dermatitis. 'Atopic' refers to a collection of diseases that are hereditary including asthma, hayfever and atopic dermatitis. Atopic dermatitis (eczema) is a chronic skin disease characterised by an itchy, dry, inflamed skin causing redness, cracking, weeping, crusting, excoriations and sometimes lichenification. Atopic dermatitis occurs most often in infants and children and its onset decreases substantially with age. Although infantile eczema is common, the condition frequently improves or enters into permanent remission in the early teens; however, many are still affected throughout their life. In infants, eczema usually presents after 6 weeks of life, commonly affecting the face, forehead, chest and extensor surfaces of the extremities. In children it usually affects the flexor surfaces, such as the antecubital and popliteal areas, as well as the face, neck, back, ankles and wrists. Eczema is associated with an increased incidence of contact dermatitis, molluscum, warts and herpetic viral infections. Primary eczema lesions can be infected by secondary staphylococcus and candida infections.

Moles and Melanomas

Malignant melanoma is an invasive malignant tumour of melanocytes. Most cases occur in white adults over the age of 30, with a predominance in women. It is the most lethal form of skin cancer. The cause is not known, but exposure to ultraviolet radiation is thought to be involved. The incidence of malignant melanoma is rising rapidly. The highest incidence of melanoma occurs in countries with the most sunshine throughout the year. However, skin type and regularity of exposure to sun are also important. Malignant melanomas may occur de novo or may develop from a pre-existing melanocytic naevus (mole). Pre-existing moles can be screened for the possible development of malignant melanomas using the ABCDE system and/or the Glasgow 7-point checklist. According to the **ABCDE** system, **A**symmetry, **B**order irregularity, **C**olour variation, **D**iameter exceeding 6 mm or **E**levation of a mole warrants further investigation. The Glasgow 7-point checklist comprises three major signs (a change in the size, shape or colour of a mole) and four minor signs (diameter exceeding 6 mm, any crusting/bleeding, inflammation or altered sensation). Patients with lesions with one major and one or more minor signs should be considered for a diagnostic excision biopsy. The only treatment of proven benefit for a malignant melanoma is surgery. An excision biopsy is recommended for all suspicious lesions. If the histology confirms the diagnosis of malignant melanoma, then a wide local excision should be performed as soon as possible. When performing a wide local excision of the malignant melanoma, a 1 cm margin of normal skin around the melanoma is removed for every millimetre of thickness up to a maximum radius of 3 cm, whereafter no extra benefit is achieved. Tissue is removed down to, but not including, the deep fascia. Histology can also be used to assess prognosis in malignant melanoma with the Breslow thickness used to calculate prognosis.

Breslow Thickness Predictive of Prognosis

The Breslow thickness is a valuable indicator when calculating the prognosis of malignant melanomas with no metastases. This is the vertical distance in millimetres from the granular cell layer of the epidermis to the deepest part of the tumour. Prognosis is calculated for 5-year survival and is dependent on the thickness of the melanoma. Overall prognosis is 62%

Thickness in mm	Prognosis (%)
< 1.5 mm	96F/91M (low risk)
> 3.5 mm	52F/42M (high risk)

4.3   DERMATOLOGY: ADVICE ON SUN PROTECTION

INSTRUCTIONS

You are a foundation year House Officer in General Practice. Mrs Cook, a 20-year-old Caucasian woman, is planning to settle in the Bahamas and work as a tourist guide. A friend of hers has recently been diagnosed with skin cancer. Counsel this patient and provide advice on sun protection and sunscreens.

INTRODUCTION

1 2 3

☐ ☐ ☐   **Introduction**   Introduce yourself. Elicit the patient's name, age and occupation. Establish rapport with the patient.

☐ ☐ ☐   **Ideas**   Elicit the patient's ideas and concerns regarding skin cancer.

'I am sorry to hear that a close friend of yours has recently been diagnosed with skin cancer. Can you tell me what you know about skin cancers?'

☐ ☐ ☐   **Concerns**   Elicit patient's concerns and explore them appropriately.

'Do you have any particular worries about skin cancer? Do you have any concerns about your new job and your chance of developing skin cancer?'

☐ ☐ ☐   **Understanding**   Check the patient's understanding of the risk of skin cancer associated with excessive sun exposure.

'What are your views on sunbathing and suntans? Do you know that too much sun exposure is not good for you? Are you aware that too much sun exposure has been linked to skin cancer? Do you know how you can protect yourself from the harmful effects of the sun?'

MEDICAL ADVICE

☐ ☐ ☐   **Sunlight**   Explain that excessive sun exposure can cause skin cancer.

'Some sunshine can be good for us, as it helps the body produce vitamin D which strengthens the bones. Sunlight has also been shown to make many of us have a feeling of well-being. However, too much sun exposure can lead to a number of skin problems, such as dryness, aging of the skin and sunburn. Sunlight is made up of different forms of energy. One in particular, ultraviolet or UV radiation, can damage the skin cells and lead to skin cancer.'

Ultraviolet (UV) Light

Ultraviolet light has a shorter wavelength than visible light and cannot be seen with the naked eye. It derives its name (Latin: *ultra* – 'beyond') from the position it holds on the electromagnetic spectrum, which is adjacent to the colour violet. It is a form of radiation that is emitted from the sun and is largely divided into three bands, UVA (long wave), UVB (medium wave) and UVC (short wave). The shorter the wavelength, the more damaging it is to the skin. The Earth's atmosphere blocks all UVC and most UVB rays. In fact, almost all radiation that penetrates through is UVA (98.7%). UVA radiation causes photo-aging whilst UVB rays cause sunburn (**mnemonic**: UV**A** – **A**ging, UV**B** – **B**urning). Both forms of radiation contribute towards the development of skin cancer

☐☐☐ **Measures**   Explain simple measures to reduce the risk of skin cancer.

Avoidance

'Most cases of skin cancer can be prevented by protecting our skin from the harmful effects of the sun. This is simple and need not be expensive. You should try to avoid sunbathing, sunbeds and tanning lamps. When you choose to go out, try to avoid the sun during its peak (from 11 am to 3 pm) when the sun's rays are strongest. If you are out in sun, avoid being out for long stretches and try to seek shade as much as possible.'

Clothing

'Ensure that you wear long sleeves and trousers rather than short sleeves and shorts. Use tightly woven clothing that will block UV radiation. Wear a wide-brimmed hat to protect your face, neck and ears. Wear a pair of UV protective sunglasses to help protect your eyes from the sun.'

☐☐☐ **Sunscreens**   Explain the role of sunscreen and the SPF and UVA system of labelling.

'Sunscreens play an important role in protecting your skin from damage by the sun's rays. However, they should not be viewed as an alternative to clothing and shade, but only as offering additional protection. It is important to note that no sunscreen will provide total protection against the sun. In addition, you should not use sunscreens to help you stay out in the sun for longer.'

'Sunscreens work by blocking out both UVA and UVB radiation so it cannot reach the skin. Sunscreens with a high level of UVA protection help defend the skin against photo-aging and potentially against skin cancer, while sunscreens with a high level of UVB protection help prevent sunburn and the skin damage that can cause skin cancer. Sunscreens that offer both UVA and UVB protection are sometimes called "broad spectrum".'

☐☐☐ *SPF*

'In the UK there are two systems of labelling sun protection products, SPF and UVA star rating. SPF stands for the sun protection factor. This indicates the amount of protection against sunburn that the sunscreen provides. The SPF system primarily shows the level of protection against UVB, not the protection against UVA. For example, using an SPF of 20 means you will receive 20 times the protection against burning, compared to not using anything.'

☐☐☐ *UVA System*

'The UVA star system ranges from zero to five stars. This informs people how effective the sunscreen is against UVA rays. The best sunscreen products will block UVA and UVB rays equally and hence will get five stars. Lower star ratings indicate that less UVA radiation is blocked in relation to UVB.'

UV Rating Star System

There is no official internationally recognised standard to measure UVA absorbance. However, in the UK, a local industry recognised standard is employed known as the UVA star rating system

Star Rating	Mean UVA: UVB ratio	Description
No stars	0.0–0.2	No sun protection offered
★	0.2–0.4	Minimum sun protection
★ ★	0.4–0.6	Moderate sun protection
★ ★ ★	0.6–0.8	Good sun protection
★ ★ ★ ★	0.8–0.9	Superior sun protection
★ ★ ★ ★ ★	> 0.9	Ultra sun protection

Recommend	Advise the patient on general characteristics of a recommended sun cream product.

'When purchasing a sunscreen, always choose one that is broad spectrum, with an SPF of 15 or above and a UVA star rating of three stars or more.'

☐☐☐ **Application**	Explain to the patient how to apply the sunscreen.

'It is important to apply sunscreen thickly and evenly over all sun-exposed areas, in particular the ears, neck, any bald patches, hands and feet. Apply sunscreen up to 30 minutes before going out in the sun, and reapply at regular intervals throughout the day.'

Forecast	Recommend that the patient should check weather forecasts before going out.

'It is important to take note of any weather reports on news bulletins. They often give a UV sunburn forecast, which gives you a good guide as to how strong the sun's rays will be on a particular day and the level of protection required.'

Ultraviolet (UV) Index

The UV index is a standardised method to measure the strength of UV (ultraviolet) radiation from the sun on a particular day. It is a scale that is used by weather forecasters to give the general public an idea of how much precaution they should take and how much protection is needed against the sun's rays.

UV index	Colour	Description
0–2	Green	No danger. Wear sunglasses
3–5	Yellow	Little risk. Sunscreen and hat
6–7	Orange	High risk. Sunscreen (SPF 15+), avoid peak hours
8–10	Red	Very high risk. Take extra precautions
> 10	Violet	Extreme risk. Take all precautions

EVALUATION

☐☐☐ **Understanding**   Confirm that the patient has understood what you have explained to them.

☐☐☐ **Questions**   Respond appropriately to the patient's questions.

☐☐☐ **Leaflet**   Offer to give them more information in the form of a handout. Advise that the leaflet contains much of the information you have mentioned.

COMMUNICATION SKILLS

☐☐☐ **Rapport**   Attempt to establish rapport with the patient through the use of appropriate eye contact.

☐☐☐ **Fluency**   Speak fluently and do not use jargon.

☐☐☐ **Summarise**   Give a brief summary to the patient about what has been discussed. Thank the patient. Conclude the consultation.

EXAMINER'S EVALUATION

1 2 3 4 5
☐☐☐☐☐ Overall assessment of sun protection advice
☐☐☐☐☐ Role player's score
Total mark out of 30

INSTRUCTIONS

You are a foundation year House Officer in General Practice. Mrs Charles is planning to go on holiday to Spain with her family and would like to know more about sunscreen and how to apply it correctly. She is particularly worried about her two young children. Explain the correct way to apply sunscreen and deal appropriately with her concerns.

INTRODUCTION

1 2 3

☐☐☐   **Introduction**   Introduce yourself. Elicit the patient's name, age and occupation. Establish rapport with the patient.

☐☐☐   **Ideas**   Elicit the patient's ideas and concerns regarding sunscreen.

'I understand that you are going on holiday and would like to know a bit more about sunscreen lotion. Can you tell me what you know about sunscreens?'

☐☐☐   **Concerns**   Elicit the patient's concerns, i.e. not knowing the correct technique of applying sunscreen and confusion over the sunscreen grading system.

'Do you have any particular concerns about applying sunscreen?'

☐☐☐   **Expectations**   Elicit the patient's expectations.

'Is there anything in particular that you would like to learn about today?'

MEDICAL ADVICE

*Sunscreens

☐☐☐   **UV Light**   Explain the dangers of excessive sun exposure.

'The sun can emit ultraviolet (UV) radiation which can potentially harm the skin and that is why it is necessary to take precautions. The types of UV light are UVA, which can damage deeper layers of the skin and cause aging and wrinkles, and UVB, which causes tanning but also burning. UVB can damage the DNA of skin cells, which can lead to skin cancer. However, it is possible to achieve good protection against it by taking precautions when going out in the sun.'

□□□ **Precautions**   Explain the necessary precautions to avoid excessive sun exposure, such as avoiding peak hours, appropriate clothing, staying in shade where possible.

'There are some simple precautions that you and your children can take from the sun. Keep yourself inside or under the shade when the sun is at its strongest, between 11 am and 3 pm. Other things you can do to protect yourself are to wear hats with wide brims, loose-fitting baggy clothes, neck protectors for children and sunglasses for UV protection. Sunscreen is an additional tool in protecting your skin from the sun's harmful rays.'

□□□ **Grade System**   Briefly explain the sun protection factor (SPF) and the UV star rating system.

'In the UK there are two systems of labelling sun protection products, SPF and UVA star rating. SPF stands for sun protection factor. The SPF system primarily shows the level of protection against UVB, not the protection against UVA. For example, using a cream with an SPF of 20 means you will receive 20 times the protection against burning, compared to using nothing. The UVA star system ranges from 0 to 5 stars. This informs people how effective the sunscreen is against UVA rays. The best sunscreen products will block UVA and UVB rays equally and hence will get five stars. Lower star ratings indicate that less UVA radiation is being blocked in relation to UVB.'

*Application

□□□ **Pre-exposure**   Give advice regarding pre-exposure application.

'Make sure that before applying the cream the skin is clean and dry. Try to apply it at least 15 minutes to half an hour before going out into the sun.'

□□□ Application   Explain the importance in applying sufficient quantities of cream.

'Most people who use sunscreen do not apply enough of it for adequate protection. This leads to increased risk of skin damage. When applying the cream, apply generous amounts to the trunk, arms, legs and face. You must also be sure not to miss out the hands, feet, neck, around the eyes, ears, lips and the head if it is shaved or bald.'

□□□ **Rule of Nines**   Explain the rule of nines principle to provide adequate coverage.

'In order to achieve full protection according to the sun protection factor stated on the cream, it is important to apply sufficient quantities of cream to the various parts of the body. This is easy if you follow the simple rule of nines. This means that the total surface area of skin is split up into 11 sections with each section representing 9% of the total. For each of these areas you must apply the same amount of cream equally. You can do this by squeezing out two strips of sunscreen cream from the palm crease of your hand to the tips of your index and middle fingers.'

The Rule of Nines

Most people fail to apply sufficient sunscreen on their body to ensure that the proper sun protection factor (SPF) is achieved. On average, due to their poor technique, people obtain only about one-third or one-quarter of the SPF stated on the product. 'The rule of nine' (a tool also used to assess skin burns) can be used to ensure adequate sun protection is applied. The body is divided into 11 areas, each area representing 9% of the total body surface area. Two strips of sun cream should be applied to the index and middle fingers and applied to each region. This will achieve an ideal thickness of sun cream over the body (2 mm thickness per every 1 cm^2 of skin).

ELEVEN AREAS OF THE BODY

1   Head, neck and face
2   Left arm
3   Right arm
4   Upper back
5   Lower back
6   Front chest
7   Front abdomen
8   Left upper leg and thigh
9   Right upper leg and thigh
10   Left lower leg and foot
11   Right lower leg and foot

☐☐☐   **Rubbing In**   Explain that the sunscreen should remain visible after rubbing in.

'Rub in the cream only lightly. The cream should remain visible even after rubbing.'

☐☐☐   **Reapply**   Explain that sunscreen should be reapplied regularly, particularly to the areas that are uncovered.

'It is important to reapply the sunscreen regularly, at 2-hour intervals to ensure adequate protection. You must always reapply it after swimming, towelling, sweating or playing in the sand. However, for children it is important to reapply every hour. Focus on the areas that are exposed, such as the neck, face, ears and arms, and do not hesitate to use generous amounts.'

☐☐☐ **Warn**   Warn that sunscreen should never be used to spend longer in the sun.

'No sunscreen will provide 100% protection against the sun. In addition, you should not believe that sunscreens will help you stay out in the sun for longer.'

Storage   Explain that sunscreen should not be stored in very hot places (above 25°C) and should not be used past its expiry date.

EVALUATION

☐☐☐ **Understanding**   Confirm that the patient has understood what you have explained to them.
☐☐☐ **Questions**   Respond appropriately to the patient's questions.
☐☐☐ **Leaflet**   Offer to give them more information in the form of a handout. Advise that the leaflet contains much of the information you have mentioned.

COMMUNICATION SKILLS

☐☐☐ **Rapport**   Attempt to establish rapport with the patient through the use of appropriate eye contact.
☐☐☐ **Fluency**   Speak fluently and do not use jargon.
☐☐☐ **Summarise**   Give a brief summary to the patient about what has been discussed. Thank the patient. Conclude the consultation.

EXAMINER'S EVALUATION

1 2 3 4 5
☐☐☐☐☐ Overall assessment of explaining sunscreen application
☐☐☐☐☐ Role player's score
          Total mark out of 35

Psychiatry

5

INSTRUCTIONS

You are in General Practice. Mrs Canington has not seen you before but has attended today as she is feeling very low and tearful. Assess her problem and psychiatric state. You will be marked on your ability to elicit an appropriate psychiatric history and to reach a diagnosis, and on your communication skills.

INTRODUCTION

1 2 3

☐☐☐ **Introduction**   Introduce yourself. Establish rapport.
☐☐☐ **Patient Details**   Elicit name, age and occupation.

THE HISTORY

☐☐☐ **Complaint**   Elicit all of the patient's presenting complaints.
☐☐☐ **History**   'When did it first start? What has been happening recently? How long has it been going on for? What do you think caused it? How has this affected you?'

CORE SYMPTOMS

☐☐☐ **Low Mood**   'Have you been depressed or feeling low in spirits recently?'
☐☐☐ **Anhedonia**   'Do you still enjoy the activities that you used to enjoy before?'
☐☐☐ **Fatigue**   'Do you feel you don't have the same amount of energy as before? Or that you tire easily?'
☐☐☐ **Cause**   'What do you think caused you to feel this way? Are there any particular stresses at work or at home which have contributed?'

COGNITIVE SYMPTOMS

☐☐☐ **Hopeless**   'How do you feel about the future? Do you feel any hope for it?'
☐☐☐ **Helpless**   'Do you feel helpless about your current situation?'
☐☐☐ **Worthless**   'How do you feel about yourself? Do you feel you are of no worth?'
☐☐☐ **Concentration**   'Are you finding it hard to concentrate when you watch TV or read?'
☐☐☐ **Self-esteem**   'Would you say you have low self-esteem?'
☐☐☐ **Guilt**   'Do you feel that you are responsible for the situation you are in?'

BIOLOGICAL SYMPTOMS

☐☐☐ **Sleep**   'How has your sleep been? Do you find yourself waking early in the morning?'

☐☐☐ **Diurnal** 'Is there a time of day when you feel particularly bad? Do you find that you feel worse in the morning and you improve as the day progresses?'

☐☐☐ **Appetite** 'Are you eating properly? Has there been any change in your appetite?'

☐☐☐ **Libido** 'How is your libido? Have you lost interest in sex?'

DIFFERENTIAL

☐☐☐ **Bipolar** 'I know you feel low now, but have you ever felt so high and energetic that others have said that you seem elated?'

☐☐☐ **Psychosis** 'Have you ever heard voices when there was no one there? Or seen something that you did not expect to see?'

SUICIDAL IDEATION

☐☐☐ **Thoughts** 'Have you ever thought about taking your own life? How often do you get these thoughts? Are you able to resist them?'

☐☐☐ **Method** 'Have you ever thought about ways of doing it?'

☐☐☐ **Attempt** 'Have you actually tried harming yourself? What stops you from doing it?'

☐☐☐ **Impact** 'Do you have any particular concerns or worries about the symptoms you are experiencing? How have these symptoms affected your life and your family?'

ASSOCIATED HISTORY

☐☐☐ **Psych History** 'Have you ever harmed yourself in the past? Have you suffered from depression in the past? Do you suffer from any chronic health problems?'

☐☐☐ **Drug History** 'Are you taking any medications? Do you have any drug allergies?'

☐☐☐ **Family History** 'Has anyone in your family suffered from depression or psychiatric illness?'

SOCIAL HISTORY

☐☐☐ **Employment** 'Current and previous or unemployed?'

☐☐☐ **Family** 'Are you single or in a relationship? Any children?'

☐☐☐ **Support** 'Friends and family?'

☐☐☐ **Smoking** 'How many, for how long?'

☐☐☐ **Alcohol** 'How much, how often?'

☐☐☐ **Recreat. Drugs** 'Do you take any drugs? Which ones?'

☐☐☐ **Insight** 'Do you think you are depressed? How would you feel about taking medications for your problem? Do you think you can be helped?'

COMMUNICATION SKILLS

☐☐☐ **Rapport** — Establish and maintain rapport and demonstrate listening skills.
☐☐☐ **Responds** — React positively to and acknowledge patient's emotions.
☐☐☐ **Fluency** — General fluency and non-use of jargon.
☐☐☐ **Summarise** — Check with patient and deliver an appropriate summary.

'This is Mrs Canington, a 30-year-old unemployed lady with one child. She has presented complaining of low mood and tearfulness for the past 3 months since losing her job as a dental assistant. Previously an outgoing person, she has found herself lying in bed feeling tired all the time. She has no interest in watching television or reading novels. She wakes at 5 am, when her mood is at its lowest. She has no previous medical or psychiatric illness. She feels guilty as she no longer is bringing any money into the household and has loss interest in sex. She has had fleeting thoughts of harming herself but as yet has not carried these out. She denies any hallucinations or abnormal delusions. The findings from the history are consistent with a presentation of depression. However, I would like to exclude bipolar disorder.'

EXAMINER'S EVALUATION

1 2 3 4 5
☐☐☐☐☐ Overall assessment of taking depressive history
☐☐☐☐☐ Role player's score
Total mark out of 36

DIFFERENTIAL DIAGNOSIS

Depression

The diagnostic criteria for depression requires the following:
Depressed mood or anhedonia for more than 2 weeks (core symptoms)
Impaired function which may manifest in social, occupational or educational difficulties
Specific symptoms (as detailed above) of which there must be at least 5
The presence of psychotic symptoms such as hallucinations or delusions (mood congruent) indicates major depressive disorder.

Differential diagnosis/depression mimics

Other psychiatric disorders	Medical illness	Substance misuse	Bereavement disorders
Bipolar disorder	Chronic illness	Alcoholism	Bereavement or prolonged grief disorder.
Schizophrenia	Terminal illness	Substance misuse	
Schizoaffective disorder			A prolonged and more severe version of the normal
Hypomania			response to bereavement.
Mania			

BIPOLAR DISORDER

Bipolar disorder consists of episodes of mania/hypomania and depression. Male and females have the same incidence of bipolar disorder, with the age of onset usually being in the 20s. One must have two episodes of mood disturbance for the diagnosis to be considered. During the elation phase the patient may appear wearing brightly coloured, ill-matched clothes. Their behaviour will often be overactive and irritable, starting many activities and leaving them unfinished, and they may be extravagant in spending money. The patient may also be disinhibited, with increased sexual desire.

Speech and thought patterns may appear erratic. In the severe form, the patient follows a pattern of rapidly changing thoughts that may be difficult to understand (flight of ideas). Persecutory delusions and grandiose delusions are most common. They almost universally display lack of insight regarding their condition.

Mnemonic for Symptoms of Mania

MNEMONIC: MANIC

Mood (irritable)/**M**outh (pressure of speech)
Activity increased, **A**ttention (distractibility)
Naughty (disinhibition)
Insomnia, **I**deas (flight of)
Confidence (grandiose ideas)

5.2   PSYCHIATRY: HALLUCINATIONS AND DELUSIONS

INSTRUCTIONS

You are in General Practice. Ms Florence has not seen you before but her parents have asked you to assess her as they are very concerned. Assess her problem and psychiatric state. You will be marked on your ability to elicit an appropriate psychiatric history, to reach a diagnosis and on your communication skills.

INTRODUCTION

1 2 3

☐☐☐   **Introduction**   Introduce yourself. Establish rapport.
☐☐☐   **Patient Details**   Elicit name, age and occupation.

THE HISTORY

☐☐☐   **Complaint**   Elicit all of the patient's presenting complaints. The key to taking a history of delusions is the same as taking a sexual history: you need to be completely non-judgemental and open in your interview technique.

☐☐☐   **History**   'When did it first start? What has been happening recently? How long has it been going on for? What do you think caused it? How has this affected you?'

DELUSIONS

☐☐☐   **Persecutory**   'Do you think people are against you? Is anyone trying to harm you?'

☐☐☐   **Grandeur**   'Do you have any special powers which other people may not have?'

☐☐☐   **Perception**   'Do you believe or understand things differently from other people?'

☐☐☐   **Reference**   'Do you get any special messages from the TV or radio?'
☐☐☐   **Nihilistic**   'Do you feel that all around you is dying and false?'
☐☐☐   **Content**   'When did you first realise this (i.e. the delusional belief) was true? How?'

☐☐☐   **Unshakeable**   'How would you feel if I were to tell you that you do not have these powers?'

HALLUCINATIONS

☐☐☐   **Auditory**   'Do you ever hear voices when no one is present?'
☐☐☐   **Real/Pseudo**   'Do the voices come from inside your head or from outside?'

☐☐☐ **2nd/3rd Person** 'Do they talk directly to you or about you? Do they comment on what you do? What do they talk about? Do they want you to harm yourself or other people?'

☐☐☐ **1st Person** 'Do you ever hear your thoughts repeated like an echo (Echo de la Pensée)?'

☐☐☐ **Visual** 'Have you ever seen things that were not there or could not explain?'

☐☐☐ **Olfactory** 'Have you smelt something that was not present?'

THOUGHT DISORDERS

☐☐☐ **Insertion** 'Have you ever felt that someone had put ideas into your head?'

☐☐☐ **Withdrawal** 'Have you ever felt that someone removed thoughts from your head?'

☐☐☐ **Broadcasting** 'Have you ever felt that other people can hear what you are thinking?'

PASSIVITY PHENOMENA

☐☐☐ **Control** 'Have you ever felt that your thoughts or actions are controlled by someone else without your will? Do they make you do things against your wishes?'

☐☐☐ **Impact on Life** 'How is all this affecting your life at the moment?'

☐☐☐ **Mood** 'What is your mood like at the moment?'

ASSOCIATED HISTORY

☐☐☐ **Psych History** 'Has this ever happened in the past before? Have you ever suffered from depression? Have you ever harmed yourself in the past? Do you have any other health problems?'

☐☐☐ **Drug History** 'Are you on any medication? Do you have any drug allergies?'

☐☐☐ **Family History** 'Has anyone in your family suffered from any psychiatric illness?'

SOCIAL HISTORY

☐☐☐ **Work** 'Are you currently working? How is your work? Any stress?'

☐☐☐ **Family** 'Are you single or in a relationship? Do you get support from friends and family? Do you have any children?'

☐☐☐ **Other** 'Do you smoke, drink alcohol or take recreational drugs?'

☐☐☐ **Insight** 'Do you think you have a problem? How would you feel about taking medications if these were deemed appropriate?'

COMMUNICATION SKILLS

☐☐☐ **Rapport** Establish and maintain rapport and demonstrate listening skills.

☐☐☐ **Responds** React positively to and acknowledge patient's emotions.

☐☐☐ **Fluency**   General fluency and non-use of jargon.
☐☐☐ **Summarise**   Check with patient and deliver an appropriate summary.

'This is Ms Florence, a 22-year-old unemployed lady who was referred by her parents who have been concerned about her suspicious behaviour. She mentions that she believes people are following her wherever she goes and she is able to predict the future from messages she receives through her TV. She mentions that she hears two voices inside her head which talk about her all the time. They do not order her to harm herself or others. She denies any visual hallucinations. With regard to her thoughts, she mentions that sometimes when she is thinking about something, someone takes thoughts out of her head. She has no previous medical or psychiatric illness and is not on any medication. She admits to "experimenting" with different recreational drugs including cocaine and cannabis recently. She denies any mood disorder.

'The findings from the history are consistent with a presentation of schizophrenia. However, I would like to exclude delusional and bipolar disorder.'

EXAMINER'S EVALUATION

1 2 3 4 5
☐☐☐☐☐ Overall assessment of taking a hallucination history
☐☐☐☐☐ Role player's score
     Total mark out of 44

DIFFERENTIAL DIAGNOSIS

Schizophrenia

Schizophrenia is a chronic, severe, disabling brain disorder. It affects men and women equally, often appearing earlier in men, during their 20s. It is largely defined by the presence of one of more of Schneider's first-rank symptoms, including delusions of perception, delusions of thought control, delusions of control/passivity and auditory hallucinations (first person or third person). Symptoms must be present for more than a month in the absence of any identifiable organic brain disease or alcoholic intoxication.

Schizophrenia subtypes

Paranoid	Catatonic	Disorganised	Undifferentiated	Residual
Dominated by delusions and hallucinations.	The finding of catatonic stupor or waxy flexibility	Dominated by thought disorder and flattened affect	Dominated by psychotic symptoms	Low-intensity positive symptoms

Delusional disorder

This group of disorders is characterised by the development of a single delusion or of a set of related delusions which persist. Although the delusions are highly variable in content, often being persecutory, hypochondriacal or grandiose, they may be concerned with litigation or jealousy. Depressive symptoms may present intermittently and olfactory and tactile hallucinations may develop in some cases (although these are rare). The delusions must be present for at least 1 month for the diagnosis to be made after organic brain disease has been excluded. They are differentiated from schizophrenia due to the absence of delusions of passivity or thought control.

Bipolar disorder

Episodes of mania with psychosis can be confused with schizophrenia. Bipolar psychosis presents as secondary delusions in response to abnormal mood. Delusions are usually mood congruent, with the content matching the mood of the person. Persecutory delusions and grandiose delusions are most common. See under depression for more details.

5.3   PSYCHIATRY: ASSESSING SUICIDE RISK

INSTRUCTIONS

You are about to see Ms Pickers, a travel agent. She was admitted last night following an overdose of 10 paracetamol tablets. She has not been started on any treatment as her overdose level was below the treatment line. Take a history from the patient and establish her suicide risk.

INTRODUCTION

1 2 3
☐☐☐ **Introduction**   Introduce yourself. Establish rapport.
☐☐☐ **Patient Details**   Elicit name, age and occupation.

THE HISTORY

☐☐☐ **Complaint**   Elicit all of the patient's presenting complaints.
☐☐☐ **History**   'How are you feeling today? What made you feel that you had to take your life? What exactly happened?'

PYSCHIATRIC SYMPTOMS BEFORE THE ATTEMPT

☐☐☐ **Before**   'What happened just before you tried ending your life? Have you been feeling low and depressed? How long for?'
☐☐☐ **Planning**   'Did you plan for this to happen? Did you go out and prepare the tablets?'
☐☐☐ **Seeking Help** 'Did you tell anybody about the attempt? Or try to get help?'
☐☐☐ **Precautions**   'Did you take any precautions against getting caught or discovered?'
☐☐☐ **Final Acts**   'Did you make a will? Or leave a note? Did you close your bank accounts?'

THE ATTEMPT

☐☐☐ **Incident**   'What did you do? How did you do it? When and where?'
☐☐☐ **Meaning**   'Did you really want to die and escape your problems?'
☐☐☐ **Fatality**   'Did you think the attempt was going to kill you?'
☐☐☐ **Discovered** 'How were you discovered?'
☐☐☐ **Alcohol**   'Were you under the influence of alcohol during the attempt?'

AFTER THE ATTEMPT

☐☐☐ **Feel**   'How do you feel now? Angry as it was not successful or regretful?'
☐☐☐ **Thoughts** 'Do you still have any lingering thoughts to take your life?'
☐☐☐ **Mood**   'Do you feel depressed? How do you see the future?'

RISK FACTORS

☐☐☐ **Home**   'Do you live alone?'

☐☐☐ **Family**   'Are you in a relationship? Do you have a husband? Any
children?'

☐☐☐ **Work**   'Are you working? Do you have any work-related stress?'

ASSOCIATED HISTORY

☐☐☐ **Psych History**   'Any previous suicide attempts? Have you ever harmed yourself
in the past? Do you have any psychiatric illnesses such as
depression, schizophrenia or mania? Do you suffer from any
of the following chronic illnesses: multiple sclerosis/cancer/
epilepsy?'

☐☐☐ **Drug History**   'Are you taking any medications? Do you have any drug
allergies?'

☐☐☐ **Family History**   'Does anyone have any psychiatric problems in your family? Has
anyone harmed themselves or tried to take their own lives?'

☐☐☐ **Social History**   'Do you drink alcohol? How much and how often? Do you
smoke? Have you ever tried any recreational drugs?'

☐☐☐ **Insight**   'Do you feel you need help? Would you accept any help if offered
to you?'

☐☐☐ **Follow-up**   Provide appropriate patient risk assessment and advise on
management, i.e. need for inpatient admission or outpatient
follow-up.

COMMUNICATION SKILLS

☐☐☐ **Rapport**   Establish and maintain rapport and demonstrate listening skills.

☐☐☐ **Responds**   React positively to and acknowledge patient's emotions.

☐☐☐ **Fluency**   General fluency and non-use of jargon.

☐☐☐ **Summarise**   Check with patient and deliver an appropriate summary.

'This is Ms Pickers, an 18-year-old travel agent. She was admitted yesterday after having
taken an overdose of 10 paracetamol tablets. She took the tablets after having an argument
with her boyfriend, who she discovered had cheated on her. This was the first time
she has tried to harm herself or take her life and she denies planning the attempt. She
mentions that she was angry and wanted to make her boyfriend "feel guilty". She feels
remorseful for what she has done and does not wish to carry it out again. She is glad that
she is well and was discovered. She lives with her parents and two siblings. She has no
previous psychiatric history nor is there any positive psychiatric family history. She denies
hallucinations, low mood or delusions. She is a non-smoker, social drinker and has not
tried any recreational drugs. She is happy to seek help and is willing to attend outpatient
follow-up clinics.'

EXAMINER'S EVALUATION

1 2 3 4 5
☐ ☐ ☐ ☐ ☐   Overall assessment of suicidal risk
☐ ☐ ☐ ☐ ☐   Role player's score
Total mark out of 35

Risk Factors for Suicide

MNEMONIC: SAD PERSONS

Sex (male)
Age (Elderly or young 19–34)
Depression
Previous attempts/FH of suicide
Ethanol abuse or other drugs
Rational thinking lost
Social support lacking (single)
Organised suicide plan
No job (unemployed/retired) or spouse
Sickness (chronic)

5.4   PSYCHIATRY: ASSESSING ALCOHOL DEPENDENCY

INSTRUCTIONS

Mr Butler is a 23-year-old law student. You have not met him before and are interviewing him in General Practice. You have noted from the records that he may have an alcohol problem but this has not yet been discussed with the patient. Assess his drinking behaviour and give some advice with appropriate follow-up.

INTRODUCTION

1 2 3

☐☐☐   **Introduction**   Introduce yourself. Establish rapport.
☐☐☐   **Patient Details**   Elicit name, age and occupation.
☐☐☐   **Explain**

'I have been asked to talk to you about your health and in particular about your drinking habits. Has anyone spoken to you about this before?'

ALCOHOL HISTORY: DRINKING HABITS

☐☐☐   **Type**   'What type of beverages do you drink? Beer, wine or spirits?'
☐☐☐   **Amount**   'How much do you drink a day? How much do you drink a week?'
☐☐☐   **Intake Pattern** 'Is there a certain time you drink? Can you tell me your typical drinking day?'
☐☐☐   **Reason**   'What causes you to drink like this?'
☐☐☐   **First Start**   'At what age did you first start to drink?'

ALCOHOL DEPENDENCE

☐☐☐   **Compulsion**   'Do you crave for alcohol when you are unable to drink?'
☐☐☐   **Primacy**   'Would you say alcohol was a priority over other aspects of your life?'
☐☐☐   **Tolerance**   'Are you drinking more alcohol to get the same effect?'
☐☐☐   **Withdrawal**   'Do you suffer symptoms when you go without alcohol for a period of time i.e. anxiety/tremors/sweating/nausea/fits or hallucinations?'
☐☐☐   **Relieved**   'Are these symptoms relieved by drinking more alcohol?'

CAGE QUESTIONNAIRE

☐☐☐   **Cut Down**   'Have you tried to cut down?'
☐☐☐   **Angry**   'Have you felt angry at the remarks of others regarding your drinking?'
☐☐☐   **Guilty**   'Have you felt guilty about how much you drink?'
☐☐☐   **Eye Opener**   'Do you ever drink first thing in the morning?'

BELIEFS ABOUT ALCOHOL

☐☐☐ **Harmful**   'Do you believe alcohol is bad for you?'

☐☐☐ **Effects**   'Do you know what effects alcohol has on your health if you drink too much?'

☐☐☐ **Impact**   'Do you have any particular concerns or worries about how much you drink? How has your drinking affected your life and your family?'

ATTEMPTS TO REDUCE ALCOHOL

☐☐☐ **Self**   'Have you ever tried to reduce your alcohol consumption?'

☐☐☐ **Organisation**   'Did you ever join an organisation to reduce your alcohol intake? How many times have you tried and how long for?'

ASSOCIATED HISTORY

☐☐☐ **Medical History**   'Have you ever had peptic ulcers, pancreatitis, raised BP or liver disease?'

☐☐☐ **Drug History**   'Are you on any medications? Are you allergic to any drugs?'

☐☐☐ **Family History**   'Did anyone in your family drink alcohol excessively?'

SOCIAL HISTORY

☐☐☐ **Stress**   'Any relationship or financial problems?'

☐☐☐ **Work**   'What do you work as? How is your work? Any stress?'

☐☐☐ **Family**   'Are you single or currently in a relationship?'

☐☐☐ **Other**   'Do you smoke or take recreational drugs?'

INSIGHT

'Do you feel you need help? Would you accept help if it was offered to you?'

DRINKING ADVICE

Amount

'The maximum weekly intake of alcohol is 14 units for women and up to 21 units for men. It seems you may be drinking an unhealthy quantity of alcohol.'

Withdrawal

'You are developing a need for alcohol, which is why you may experience withdrawal symptoms like anxiety, sweating, tremors and blackouts.'

Damage

'Alcohol damages the brain leading to fits and memory loss; it damages the heart and liver and increases the chance of oesophageal cancer.'

Cut Down

'I strongly recommend you do your utmost to cut down. Alcohol can put pressure on relationships with your partner, family and friends, and can lead to difficulties at work and financial strain.'

Social Habits

'To cut down, try pacing your drinking when out. Buy non-alcoholic drinks between alcoholic drinks to slow the rate at which you drink. If you are going to buy the rounds, buy them but do not buy one for yourself.'

Groups

'We can put you in touch with help groups like Alcoholics Anonymous, who are experts in helping you deal with alcohol. How would you feel about this?'

COMMUNICATION SKILLS

☐☐☐ **Rapport**   Establish and maintain rapport and demonstrate listening skills.
☐☐☐ **Responds**   React positively to and acknowledge patient's emotions.
☐☐☐ **Fluency**   General fluency and non-use of jargon.
☐☐☐ **Summarise** Check with patient and deliver an appropriate summary.

'This is Mr Butler, a 23-year-old law student. He admits to drinking a lot more than his peers. He has been drinking since he was 16 and his habit has been increasing. He drinks all types of alcohol from beer to spirits depending on how he feels. He typically wakes up at 6 am and has a shot of vodka; he then spends the rest of the day looking for money so that he can buy some cans of beer from the local shop. At lunch he drinks 3 cans of beer and does not eat any food. He demonstrates tolerance and withdrawal symptoms if he does not drink alcohol. He has previously attended Alcoholics Anonymous on two occasions for 1 month. He denies any medical problems or psychiatric conditions. He wishes to come off alcohol as it is causing strains on the relationship with his parents and girlfriend. He has also been threatened with redundancy from his part-time job.'

EXAMINER'S EVALUATION

1 2 3 4 5
☐☐☐☐☐ Overall assessment of alcohol consumption and advice
☐☐☐☐☐ Role player's score
Total mark out of 45

5.5 PSYCHIATRY: ASSESSING MENTAL STATE

INSTRUCTIONS

Mr Peerman is a 43-year-old shop assistant. You have not met him before and are interviewing him in General Practice. Ask him the relevant questions to assess his mental state.

INTRODUCTION

1 2 3

☐ ☐ ☐ **Introduction**   Introduce yourself. Establish rapport.

☐ ☐ ☐ **Patient Details**   Elicit name, age and occupation.

☐ ☐ ☐ **Explain**

'I am here today to speak to you about your health and in particular about your state of mind. Will it be OK for me to ask you some questions?'

OBSERVATION: APPEARANCE AND BEHAVIOUR

☐ ☐ ☐ **Appearance**   Inspect patient's clothes. Is he well dressed or inappropriately dressed? Look to the patient's posture and facial expression. Any signs of self-neglect, i.e. unshaven, dishevelled?

☐ ☐ ☐ **Activity**   Assess the patient's activity. Is he underactive or overactive? Is he excitable or restless? Is he agitated or tearful? Does he look retarded and slow?

☐ ☐ ☐ **Behaviour**   How is the patient behaving? Is he apathetic and withdrawn? Or is he suspicious, irritable or agitated?

SPEECH

☐ ☐ ☐ **Articulation**   Does the patient have problems with articulating speech (dysarthria)?

☐ ☐ ☐ **Rate**   Is the patient's speech pressured and accelerated? Or slow with long pauses and showing retardation?

☐ ☐ ☐ **Tone and Amount**   Is the speech monotonous or spontaneous? Is the amount of speech increased or restricted (poverty of speech)?

☐ ☐ ☐ **Form**   Does what the patient says make sense? Or is there no association between what is being said? Does he leap from one subject to another with tenuous associations (flight of ideas)? Are the subjects linked together through chance soundings of words rather than their meanings (clang associations)?

AFFECT AND MOOD

☐ ☐ ☐ **Affect**   How does the patient's mood seem objectively? Is it blunt or flat?

☐☐☐ **Mood**   'How do you feel? Is your mood low and depressed? Or high, excited and elated?'

☐☐☐ **Biological**   'Have you noticed any change (increase or decrease) to your sleep, appetite, weight or sexual desire?'

☐☐☐ **Cognitive**   'How do view your situation? Do you feel hopeless and helpless? How do you view yourself? Do you feel worthless or have low self-esteem? Do you feel on top of the world? Do you feel you can do whatever you wish?'

☐☐☐ **Anxiety**   'Have you experienced any of the following symptoms: fear, avoidance or agitation? Or have you had any recent panic attacks, feeling sweaty, palpitations, headaches or suffering with pins and needles?'

SUICIDAL INTENT

☐☐☐ **Ideas**   'Have you ever thought about killing yourself?'

☐☐☐ **Intent**   'Did you formulate a plan? How did you intend to carry it out?'

☐☐☐ **Self-harm**   'Have you ever harmed yourself in the past?'

THOUGHT CONTENT

☐☐☐ **Ideas**   'Are there any ideas in your head which you consistently think about? Is there anything that preoccupies your mind that is of concern to you?'
Document any preoccupations and other overvalued ideas.

☐☐☐ **Phobias**   'Are there any objects, circumstances or places that you would prefer that you were not near? Do you feel anxious or experience palpitations when you are close to such things?'
Document any phobic stimuli, effect of related stimuli, psychological or physiological reaction and avoidance behaviour.

☐☐☐ **Obsessions**   'Are there any actions which you find yourself repeating throughout the day?'
Document and list obsessional ideas, establishing fears (illness, fear of causing harm and contamination), behaviours (checking, cleaning, counting and dressing), perception (self-image) and impact on life.

☐☐☐ **Delusions**   'Do you think people are against you? Do you have any special powers which the average person might not have? Do you get any special messages from the TV or radio?'

PERCEPTION

☐☐☐ **Hallucinations** 'Do you see things that are not there? Or do you hear voices from objects or persons that are not present?'
If auditory hallucination, ascertain number of voices and if in 1st, 2nd or 3rd person.

☐☐☐ **Self-Awareness** 'How do your feel about yourself? Do you feel when you look in the mirror that you don't think you are connected with the person you see (depersonalisation)? Do you feel that you are detached from the world around you (derealisation)?'

ASSOCIATED HISTORY

☐☐☐ **Psych History** 'Do you have any psychiatric disorders? Do you suffer from any medical illnesses?'

☐☐☐ **Drug History** 'Are you on any medications? Do you have any drug allergies?'

☐☐☐ **Family History** 'Does anyone have any psychiatric problems in your family? Has anyone harmed themselves or tried to take their own lives?'

☐☐☐ **Social History** 'Do you drink alcohol? How much and how often? Do you smoke? Have you ever tried any recreational drugs?'

☐☐☐ **Insight** 'Do you feel you need help? Would you accept any help if offered to you?'

COMMUNICATION SKILLS

☐☐☐ **Rapport** Establish and maintain rapport and demonstrate listening skills.

☐☐☐ **Responds** React positively to and acknowledge patient's emotions.

☐☐☐ **Fluency** General fluency and non-use of jargon.

☐☐☐ **Summarise** Check with patient and deliver an appropriate summary.

EXAMINER'S EVALUATION

1 2 3 4 5

☐☐☐☐☐ Overall assessment of patient's mental state

☐☐☐☐☐ Role player's score

Total mark out of 39

5.6   PSYCHIATRY: COGNITIVE STATE EXAMINATION

INSTRUCTIONS

Mr Carter is complaining of increased memory loss and forgetfulness. You are his GP and are aware that his wife is concerned because he leaves the cooker on. Take a history to establish if he is aware of the problem and assess his mental state. Formulate a management plan and present this to the examiner.

INTRODUCTION

1 2 3
☐ ☐ ☐ **Introduction**   Appropriate introduction and establish rapport.
☐ ☐ ☐ **Patient Details**   Elicit patient's name and age.

THE HISTORY

☐ ☐ ☐ **Problems**   Elicit the patient's awareness of his forgetfulness and memory loss. Elicit the patient's concerns regarding this problem.

☐ ☐ ☐ **Explain**

'I am going to ask you a series of questions and request you to carry out a number of commands to assess your mental state. The commands may appear a little silly but we routinely ask all our patients these.'

MENTAL STATE EXAMINATION

NOTE: The Mini-Mental State Examination is assessed out of a total of 30 points. A score of 23–25 or below suggests cognitive impairment. A score of 16 or below suggests dementia. Assessing long-term memory is not part of the MMSE, but is often included as part of the OSCE assessment.

ORIENTATION

☐ ☐ ☐ **Person**   'What is your name? How old are you?'
☐ ☐ ☐ **Time**   'What is the year/season/month/day/date?'
☐ ☐ ☐ **Space**   'What country/county/city/building/floor are we in/on?'

REGISTRATION

☐ ☐ ☐ **Short-term Mmry.**   Name three common objects (e.g. apple, ball, table) and ask the patient to repeat them. 1 point for each correct answer. Repeat them up to six times until all three are remembered.
☐ ☐ ☐ **Long-term Mmry.**   Semantic: 'How do you bake a cake? How do you drive a car?'
☐ ☐ ☐ **Episodic**   'Name the dates of World Wars 1 and 2. State the name of the present Queen or Prime Minister.'

ATTENTION AND CALCULATION

☐☐☐ **Serial 7s**   Ask the patient to subtract 7 from 100 repeatedly up to five times (93, 86, 79, 72, 65) or…

☐☐☐ **Spelling**   Ask the patient to spell the word WORLD backwards (DLROW).

RECALL

☐☐☐ **3 Objects**   Ask the patient to recall the three earlier objects.

LANGUAGE

☐☐☐ **Naming**   Name these objects (show a watch and a pencil). If impaired: nominal dysphasia, dominant posterior temporal-parietal lobe lesion.

☐☐☐ **Repeating**   Repeat after me: 'No ifs, ands or buts.' If repetition impaired: Conduction aphasia interruption of traffic between Broca's and Wernicke's.

READING AND WRITING

☐☐☐ **Reading**   Ask the patient to read and obey the sentence: 'Close your eyes.'

☐☐☐ **Writing**   Ask if they can write a short sentence.

THREE-STAGE COMMAND

☐☐☐ **Command**   Ask the patient to take the piece of paper with their left hand, fold it in half and place it on the floor.

CONSTRUCTION

☐☐☐ **Drawing**   Request the patient to copy the following drawing (constructional apraxia).

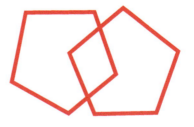

COMMUNICATION SKILLS

☐☐☐ **Rapport**   Establish and maintain rapport and demonstrate listening skills.

☐☐☐ **Fluency**   General fluency and non-use of jargon.

☐☐☐ **Summarise**   Check with patient and deliver appropriate summary.

EXAMINER'S EVALUATION

1 2 3 4 5
☐ ☐ ☐ ☐ ☐   Overall assessment of cognitive state examination
☐ ☐ ☐ ☐ ☐   Role player's score
Total mark out of 30

DIFFERENTIAL DIAGNOSIS

Dementia

Dementia is an irreversible, progressively deteriorating illness that is characterised by global impairment of cognitive function and personality without impairment to consciousness. Diagnosis is reached when symptoms persist for more than 6 months. Common symptoms of dementia include amnesia (impaired memory, especially short-term), aphasia (impaired written or verbal communication), apraxia (inability to perform simple motor movements such as in everyday tasks, e.g. dressing, eating) and agnosia (inability to recognise familiar objects or people). Dementia sufferers also display asocial behaviours and personality changes, becoming socially withdrawn and introverted or socially disinhibited. Extreme cases may also result in psychosis and the experience of hallucinations (usually visual) and delusions (persecutory).

Delirium

Delirium is characterised by disturbances of consciousness in addition to changes to attention, perception, thinking, memory, psychomotor behaviour, emotion and the sleep–wake cycle. It may occur at any age but is most common after the age of 60 years. Characteristically it has a rapid onset, with diurnal fluctuations lasting less than 6 months. Symptoms include impairment to consciousness, ranging from general clouding of consciousness to coma, and impairment to attention, with reduced ability to focus and shift attention, making patients easily distracted. There is also a global disturbance of cognition with short-term memory and recent memory impairment but with preservation of remote memory. This often leaves the patient disoriented with regard to time, place and person. Language is often affected with incoherent speech and impaired ability to understand. Other key features of delirium include perceptual distortions, ranging from misinterpretations and illusions to visual hallucinations, as well as psychomotor disturbances, ranging from under- to hyperactivity with an enhanced startle reaction. Delirious patients often suffer from mood disturbances, with bouts of depression, anxiety, irritability, euphoria and apathy as well as sleep–wake cycle disturbances ranging from disturbed sleep and insomnia to reversal of the sleep–wake cycle, including daytime drowsiness, disturbing dreams or nightmares.

Orthopaedics

6

6.1   ORTHOPAEDICS: BACK EXAMINATION

INSTRUCTIONS

Examine this patient who is complaining of sudden-onset back pain whilst gardening. Report your findings to the examiner as you go along, and make an appropriate diagnosis.

HISTORY

1 2 3

□□□ **Introduction**   Introduce yourself. Elicit the patient's name, age and occupation. Establish rapport with the patient.

*History of Presenting Complaint

History   'When did it first start? Have you had this problem in the past? Have you ever fallen or injured your back before? Were you carrying or lifting anything heavy at the time?'

□□□ **Pain**   'Where is the pain located? Does the pain move? How severe is the pain graded out of 10? Did it come on suddenly or gradually? What does the pain feel like?'

Severe pain radiating to a well-defined area with motor, sensory and reflex impairment is suggestive of a prolapsed disc. A radiating pain that is vague, diffuse and with an ill-defined distribution is most likely referred pain.

□□□ **Stiffness**   'Do you have any stiffness? Is it worse in the morning or evening? Does it come on suddenly or gradually?'

Deformity   'Have you noticed a change in the shape of your back or neck?'

□□□ **Neurology**   'Do you have weakness in your arms (cervical compression) or legs (ask about saddle anaesthesia – cauda equina)? Have you noticed any tingling or numbness in your toes or fingers? Have you noticed any problems with your bladder or bowel (urinary incontinence – spinal cord compression, retention/bowel incontinence – cauda equina lesion)?'

□□□ **General Health**   'How is your general health? Do you have any malaise, fever or weight loss?'

□□□ **Impact on Life**   'How has your back problem affected your daily activities and/or mobility?'

EXAMINATION

Consent   Explain the examination to the patient and seek their consent.

□□□ **Expose**   Ask the patient if they can undress to their undergarments.

*Gait

□□□ **Walk**   Ask to examine the patient's gait. Ask the patient if they could walk to the end of the room and return.

Signs to Look for in Gait

Use of a walking aid	Sticks, frames
Speed	Rhythm, presence of a limp
Phases of walking	Heel strike, stance, push off and swing
Stride length	Reduced, limited
Arm swing	Present, absent

*Look

☐☐☐ **Inspect**   Inspect the patient's back while they are standing. Observe the skin, shape and posture.

Signs to Observe in the Back Examination

Skin	Scars, sinus, pigmentation, abnormal hair (spina bifida), unusual skin creases
Muscle	Wasting (paravertebral, gluteal muscles), fasciculations
Posture	Observe from the back:
	List: Lateral deviation of the spine
	Scoliosis: Lateral curvature of the spine
	Observe from the side:
	Kyphosis: Undue bending of the spine
	Kyphos: Sharp bend of the spine
	Spondylolisthesis: Loss of lumbar lordosis
	Hyperlordosis: Hollowing of the lumbar spine
Asymmetry	Chest, trunk or pelvis (may appear with patient leaning forwards)

*Feel

☐☐☐ **Palpate**   Palpate the full length of the spine over the spinous processes, paravertebral muscles and interspinous ligaments for any tenderness. Establish the site of the pain.

*Move

        Movement   Ask the patient to replicate your movements. Note any limited range of movement or the citing of pain during a movement.

        Extension   Stand behind the patient and ask them to lean backwards as far as they can.

☐☐☐ *Flexion*   Ask the patient to touch their toes while keeping their knees straight.

☐☐☐ *Lateral Flexion*   Ask the patient to slide their right hand down their right leg. Repeat on the other side.

☐☐☐ *Rotation*   Fix the patient's pelvis with your hands and then ask them to rotate their chest from side to side.

        Expansion   Assess chest expansion by measuring chest circumference in full expiration and then in full inspiration. Normal expansion is around 7 cm; less than 5 cm suggests ankylosing spondylitis.

*Special Tests

☐☐☐ **Schober's Test**   Make a mark at the level of the dimples of Venus. Next make another mark 10 cm above and 5 cm below this level (a total distance of 15 cm). Ask the patent to flex their back and measure the distance from the initial top point down to the bottom point. The total distance should be greater than 20 cm (an increase of less than 5 cm is abnormal).

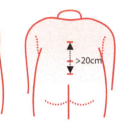

Schober's test

Make a mark at the level of dimple of Venus. Place one finger 5 cm below this mark and another finger 10 cm above this mark. Instruct the patient to flex their back. Note an increase in distance between the two fingers. An increase less than 5 cm is suggestive of a limitation of lumbar flexion.

☐☐☐ **SLR Test**   Offer assistance to get the patient onto the couch to carry out this test. Ask the patient to lie on their back keeping their legs straight. Raise the patient's leg off the couch until the patient experiences pain. Pain is commonly experienced in the thigh, buttock or back (back pain suggestive of central disc prolapse, leg pain lateral disc prolapse). Note the angle at which this occurs and then repeat the test for both legs. Normal range of movement for hip flexion is about 90° (however, 70–120° is acceptable).

The test is positive if the patient experiences pain on the affected side within the sciatic distribution between 30° and 70° of passive flexion. Pain elicited before 30° is not due to disc prolapse as the lumbar nerve roots are only brought to tension between 30° and 70°. Severe impingement (large disc herniation, central disc prolapse with cauda equina) is suggested if the patient complains of pain on the affected side when the SLR test is performed on the opposite unaffected leg (crossed sciatic reflex).

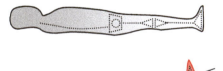

Normal

Ask the patient to lie completely flat on their back with their legs straight.

Sciatic Stretch test

Patient is unable to raise their leg beyond a certain angle due to the tension on the root by the prolapsed disc.

☐☐☐ **Bragard's Test**   If the straight-leg-raising test is positive, lower the leg on the affected side until the pain is diminished and then dorsiflex the patient's foot. If the pain is regenerated, this suggests sciatic neuritis.

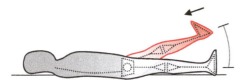

Bragard's Test

Determine the angle of hip flexion where the patient feels pain and paraesthesia. Lower the leg until the pain disappears and then gently dorsiflex the foot increasing the tension on the nerve root.

Lasègue's Test Ascertain the limit of straight leg raising that generates the pain. Next flex the knee to reduce the pressure on the sciatic nerve root which should in turn reduce the pain. Now continue to flex the hip with the knee flexed. Slowly and gently extend the knee until the pain is reproduced.

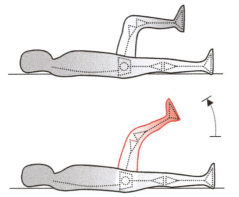

Reduce root tension

With the knee flexed, the hip is able to be elevated to a higher angle compared with the straight-leg-raising test without the pain being reproduced.

Lasègue's test

From the above position, extending the knee reproduces the sciatic pain caused by the prolapsed disc.

Bowstring Test Ask permission to perform the bowstring test. Once again, ascertain the angle of hip flexion required to generate the pain. Flex the knee slightly to relieve the pain. Next, apply firm pressure to the popliteal fossa behind the lateral hamstrings over the stretched common peroneal nerve. Induction of pain suggests nerve root irritation.

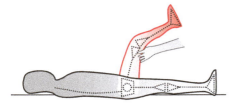

Bowstring test

Note the angle of hip flexion that causes pain. Flex the knee slightly to reduce the pain. Apply pressure with your thumb in the popliteal fossa to regenerate pain.

Femoral Stretch Ask permission to perform the femoral stretch test. Ask the patient to lie on their front. Lift the patient's leg flexing the patient's knee whilst extending the hip. A positive test suggests ipsilateral irritation of L2, L3, L4 due to a prolapsed disc.

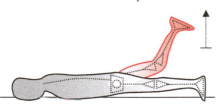

Femoral Stretch test

Ask the patient to lie prone. Flex the knee to put tension on the femoral roots and to replicate the pain. If there is no pain, slowly extend the hip with the knee flexed.

Sacroiliac Joint	Ask permission to perform the Gaenslen's test and FABER test to assess sacroiliac joint involvement (sacroiliitis – ankylosing spondylitis).
Gaenslen's Test	Have the patient lying on their back with one leg hanging off the edge of the examining couch. The opposite knee should be flexed towards the patient's chest. Push apart the patient's knees by pushing the flexed knee towards the patient's chest and the contralateral knee towards the floor. With one hip joint flexed maximally and the opposite hip joint extended, both sacroiliac joints are stressed simultaneously. Pain represents a positive test and suggests sacroiliitis.
FABER Test	Flex the hip and knee and then abduct and externally rotate the hip as far as possible so that the legs form a figure-4 shape. Next apply firm downward pressure on the protruding knee. Pain generated in the back suggests sacroiliitis.

The FAbER Test

Mnemonic: **F**lexion, **Ab**duction, **E**xternal **R**otation of the hip

---

☐☐☐	**Neurovascular**	Check capillary refill time on both feet. Check for the presence of peripheral pulses (femoral, popliteal, post-tibial and dorsalis pedis). Assess power, light touch and tendon reflexes of the legs, comparing both sides.
☐☐☐	**Request**	State that you would like to carry out a full examination of the lower limbs (neurovascular and orthopaedic) and that you would like to examine the upper limbs including the neck, shoulder and wrist.
☐☐☐	**Summarise**	Thank the patient and offer to assist them to put on their clothes. Acknowledge the patient's concerns. Summarise your findings to the examiner.

'Mr Farmer is a 57-year-old builder who was working in his garden carrying some compost. He felt a sudden sharp pain in his back that radiated to his big toe. He is complaining of persistent lower back pain, worse on lifting and bending. There are no red flag features. On examination, he has an antalgic gait and was unable to weight bear fully on the right side. His back was tender on palpation at the L5/S1 level. He also was found to have limited forward flexion and a positive SLR on the right side. Both Bragard's and Lasègue's test were positive. There were no neurovascular signs. In conclusion, I suspect that this is a case of sciatica. However, I would like to exclude malignancy or mechanical back pain.'

EXAMINER'S EVALUATION

1 2 3 4 5
☐ ☐ ☐ ☐ ☐   Overall assessment of back examination
☐ ☐ ☐ ☐ ☐   Role player's score
Total mark out of 32

DIFFERENTIAL DIAGNOSIS

Ankylosing Spondylitis

Ankylosing spondylitis is derived from the Greek word *ankylos*, meaning 'stiffening of a joint' and *spondylos*, meaning 'vertebra'. It is a generalised chronic inflammatory disease that affects predominantly the sites of insertion of ligaments and tendons in bones. It often affects the spine and sacroiliac joints but may also involve the hip, knees and smaller joints. It typically affects young males (5:1), with peak onset between 15 to 30 years, but is rarely seen to develop beyond the age of 40. It has a strong genetic component with familial inheritance and a strong association with the HLA-B27 genotype. The presenting complaint is often lower back pain and stiffness that may radiate to the buttocks. Rest does not resolve the pain but exercise and activity may improve it. The pain is noted to be worst in the morning but improves throughout the day. On examination, there is tenderness over the sacroiliac joints (sacroiliitis), loss of lumbar lordosis, increased kyphosis, reduced spinal flexion, fixed flexion of the hips and limitations in chest expansion. This often forms a classical appearance of ankylosing spondylitis. Other features include Achilles tendonitis and plantar fasciitis. Non-articular features include iritis, aortic incompetence and apical lung fibrosis.

Features of Ankylosing Spondylitis

MNEMONIC: 7 As FOR ANKYLOSING SPONDYLITIS

Achilles tendonitis
Atlantoaxial subluxation
Aortic regurgitation
Arthritis
Apical lung fibrosis
Anterior uveitis
Ig**A** nephropathy

Prolapsed Disc

A prolapsed disc is a common cause of severe lower back pain. The prolapsed disc often presses upon a nerve root which causes the pain and symptoms in the lower leg. The most common sites include the L4/5 and L5/S1 disc areas. The patient may complain of back pain when he or she lifts a heavy object while being unable to straighten their back thereafter. This can be accompanied with sciatic leg pain (sciatica) characterised by severe pain localised in the lumbar region or pain that radiates from the lower spine down the back of either leg. Both the back pain as well as sciatica can be reproduced by coughing, sneezing or straining. Other features include the presence of a list to one side, a limitation of spinal forward flexion and extension of the back with tenderness of the lower vertebrae and paravertebral muscles. The straight-leg-raising test is an important test in checking for a prolapsed disc and is limited on the affected side. Both Bragard's test and Lasègue's test can be used to confirm the diagnosis of a prolapsed disc. There are a number of neurological signs that, if identified, permit the examiner to localise the level of the prolapsed disc. Weakness of the hallux extension with loss of sensation on the outer aspect of the leg and the dorsum of the foot suggests an L4/L5 level prolapse. Pain in the calf, weakness of plantar flexion and eversion of the foot, loss of sensation over the lateral aspect of the foot and a depressed ankle reflex suggests an L5/S1 level prolapse.

Scoliosis

Scoliosis is defined as a lateral curvature of the spine, the presence of which is abnormal. The most common type of spinal curvature is idiopathic scoliosis. Idiopathic scoliosis may either be of early onset, arising before the age of seven, or late onset, after the age of seven. As much as 80% of late-onset idiopathic scoliosis occurs in girls while 80% of this group have their rib prominence on the right-hand side. The spinal curvature can bend towards either side of the body and at any place. Scoliosis can be subdivided by the location where the spine bends, i.e. in the chest area (thoracic scoliosis), in the lower part of the back (lumbar), or above and below these areas (thoraco-lumbar). If there are two bends present in the spine, it will cause an S-shaped curve (double curvature). Such an arrangement may be unnoticeable since the two curves may appear to counteract each other, leading to the appearance that the patient's back is straight and normal.

Kyphosis

Kyphosis is derived from the Greek word *kyphos*, meaning 'a hump'. It is used to describe the normal curvature of the upper spine as well as being used to describe excessive dorsal curvature. Scheuermann's disease is a form of kyphosis that occurs predominantly in teenagers. It is caused by a growth disorder of the spine whereby the vertebrae become irregular and wedge-shaped and can herniate over at least three adjacent levels. Consequently the deformity is fixed and cannot be compensated for by changes in posture as in postural kyphosis. Clinical features include fatigability and backache, which can be aggravated by strenuous exercise and long periods of sitting or standing.

6.2   ORTHOPAEDICS: SHOULDER EXAMINATION

INSTRUCTIONS

Please examine this patient with shoulder pain. Report your findings to the examiner as you go along, and make an appropriate diagnosis.

HISTORY

1 2 3

☐☐☐ **Introduction**   Introduce yourself. Elicit the patient's name, age and occupation. Establish rapport with the patient.

*History of Presenting Complaint

☐☐☐ **Pain**   'Where is the pain located? Does the pain move anywhere? What does the pain feel like? How severe is the pain graded out of 10? What were you doing at the time it started?'

Stiffness   'Do you have any stiffness? Did it come on progressively or suddenly? Is it worse in the morning or the evening?'

Swelling   'Have you noticed any swelling? Did it occur after an injury?'

☐☐☐ **Impact on Life**   'How has your shoulder problem affected your daily activities? Do you have any difficulties with dressing or grooming?'

EXAMINATION

Consent   Obtain consent before beginning the examination.

☐☐☐ **Expose**   Ask the patient if they can remove their outer garments to expose their upper body.

*Look

☐☐☐ **Inspect**   Inspect the patient from the front, behind and sides. Observe the shoulder for any obvious abnormal posture, deformity or wasting.

Signs to Inspect for in the Shoulder Examination

Alignment	Asymmetry of the shoulders, winging of the scapula
Position	Internal rotation of the arm (posterior dislocation of shoulder)
Bones	Bony prominences of the acromioclavicular joints (ACJ) and the sternoclavicular joints (SCJ), deformity of clavicle (old fracture)
Skin	Colour (bruising), sinuses, scars
Muscles	Wasting of deltoids (axillary nerve palsy), supra and infraspinatus, pectoral muscles
Axilla	Lumps (lymph), large joint effusions

*Feel

	Skin	Run the back surface of your fingers over the patient's shoulder to assess the temperature. Compare both sides.
☐☐☐	**Joints**	Palpate the shoulder for tenderness and effusions. Begin at the sternoclavicular joint then move along the clavicle towards the acromioclavicular joint, ending at the acromion. Palpate the greater and lesser tuberosities and also the glenohumeral joint. Note any tender sites.
☐☐☐	**Tendons**	Have the patient sitting with their arms straightened. Ask the patient to flex their arm, contracting the biceps muscles. Palpate the biceps tendon within the bicipital groove in an attempt to elicit pain which may suggest biceps tendonitis.

*Move

☐☐☐	**Active**	Request the patient to perform a number of active movements, including abduction, adduction, flexion, extension and rotation. Note any limited range of movements or the reporting of pain.
☐☐☐	*Abduction*	Ask the patient to raise both arms, starting from their sides and meeting above their head in the midline (180°). If pain is present, establish the angle when it begins within the painful arc. If pain occurs in the mid-range of the arc, it suggests supraspinatus tendonitis or a partial rotator cuff tear. If the pain is established at the end of the arc it may suggest acromioclavicular joint arthritis.

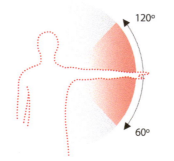

120°

60°

Painful Shoulder Arc

The 'painful arc' lies between 60 and 120 degrees of shoulder abduction. Pain noted in this arc suggests supraspinatus tendonitis or a partial rotator cuff tear.

Causes of Painful Shoulder Arc

Partial tear of supraspinatus tendon	Supraspinatus tendonitis
Calcified deposits in supraspinatus tendon	Subacromial bursitis
Fracture of greater tuberosity of humerus	

☐☐☐	*Adduction*	Ask the patient to move their arms inwards towards the midline and across their chest (50°).
☐☐☐	*Flexion*	Ask the patient to raise their arms forward (165°).
☐☐☐	*Extension*	Ask the patient to swing their arms backwards (65°).
☐☐☐	*Rotation*	To test for external rotation, have the elbows flexed at 90° and placed firmly against their sides with their hands facing

forwards. Externally rotate the shoulder by turning the arms laterally as far as possible (normal range 60°).

☐☐☐ **Scratch Test**   Perform Apley's scratch test by asking the patient to scratch their scapula with their fingers by reaching behind their back (internal rotation with adduction) and behind their neck (external rotation with abduction).

Passive   Stand behind the patient, rest one hand on their shoulder and move their arm in all planes. Observe for crepitus, pain and limitation of movement.

*Neurology

☐☐☐ **Power**   Test the deltoid muscles by asking the patient to raise their arms like wings and to hold them in position against resistance (C5/6, axillary nerve). Pectoralis major can be tested by requesting the patient to push their hands against their waist. Test the biceps by asking the patient to flex the elbow against resistance. Ask the patient to push against the wall as hard as possible to test for serratus anterior muscle (long thoracic nerve C5–7). Observe from behind for winging of the scapula.

☐☐☐ **Sensation**   Test light touch and proprioception on the upper limbs. Note any sensation loss or paraesthesia over the shoulder, particularly over the deltoid muscle, which could indicate an anterior dislocation of the shoulder.

*Special Tests

☐☐☐ **Apprehension**   The apprehension test assesses for anterior dislocation of the shoulder and can be tested in a number of ways. Have the patient in the supine position, with the arm abducted 90° and hanging off the bed. Grasp their elbow in your hand and gently rotate the shoulder externally by pushing the forearm posteriorly. At the same time, push the head of the humerus anteriorly with your other hand. Instability will give the sense that the humeral head is about to slip out anteriorly and the patient resists further movement.

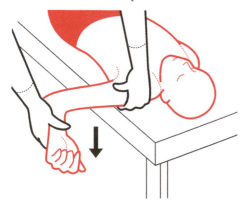

Apprehension Test

Have the patient's arm abducted to 90 degrees while lying on the edge of a couch. Hold the elbow and gently push the forearm posteriorly. Gently push the head of the humerus anteriorly with your other hand. The patient will sense that his shoulder will dislocate and resist further movement.

Alternatively, stand behind the patient with the elbow at 90°. Slowly abduct, externally rotate and extend the shoulder with one hand while applying pressure over the head of the humerus (from behind) with the opposite thumb. The patient will apprehend that their shoulder may dislocate and resist further movement.

☐☐☐ **Neer's Test**

Have the patient seated before performing Neer's impingement test. Place one hand on the patient's scapula, and grasp their forearm with your other. Internally rotate the arm with the thumb facing downwards and gently abduct and forward flex the arm. If impingement is present, the patient will experience pain as the arm is abducted. A positive test suggests subacromial impingement.

Request

State that you would also like to perform a full neck, back and elbow orthopaedic examination.

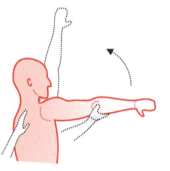

Neer's Impingement Test

Place a hand on the patient's scapula while holding their forearm with the other. Have the arm internally rotated so that the thumb is pointing downward. Next, gently forward-flex the arm up to the vertical position. A positive test is noted if the patient complains of pain.

☐☐☐ **Summarise**

Thank the patient. Acknowledge the patient's concerns. Restore the patient's clothing. Summarise your findings to the examiner.

'This is Mr Patel, a grocery shop manager, who is complaining of shoulder pain with stiffness for the last 4 months. The pain initially began after he fell off his stepladder while he was stacking shelves. The pain gradually worsened over the last few months and now he is unable to work. On examination, there is diffuse tenderness around the glenohumeral joint, and generalised reduced movement in the elbow with limited abduction and external rotation. I suspect that this patient suffers from a frozen shoulder.'

EXAMINER'S EVALUATION

1 2 3 4 5
☐☐☐☐☐ Overall assessment of shoulder examination
☐☐☐☐☐ Role player's score
Total mark out of 31

DIFFERENTIAL DIAGNOSIS

Chronic Tendinitis (Impingement Syndrome)

Impingement syndrome is a condition that affects the rotator cuff, causing shoulder pain. Impingement of the rotator cuff muscles against the coracoacromial ligament is believed to be the cause of this condition. Impingement occurs due to repetitive overhead activities such as swimming, skiing, tennis or jobs involving reaching high up. Symptoms include pain and weakness. Pain originates in the shoulder and over the deltoid muscle and is exacerbated by above-the-head activities. A frequent complaint is night pain, often disturbing sleep, particularly when the patient lies on the affected shoulder. Weakness and loss of motion are associated symptoms. On examination the impingement tests described above are invariably positive. There is a painful arc between 60° and 120° of abduction. However, this is usually absolved if the patient repeats abduction with the arm in full external rotation.

Cervical Radiculopathy

Cervical radiculopathy is nerve root dysfunction in the cervical spine in which symptoms are generated from nerve root compression. It is often caused by a herniated disc (young), degenerative disc disease (old) or acute injury (whiplash). Most commonly C6 and C7 are affected. Symptoms include pain, numbness and weakness affecting different areas depending on the involvement of the nerve root. Patients often describe a diffuse shoulder pain that ranges from a dull ache to a burning pain. As the condition progresses, the pain may radiate to the medial border of the scapula, occiput, arm or hand. Neck pain is frequently absent. On examination, there is reduced range of movement in the neck, with extension and neck rotation generating the pain. There is loss of sensation, muscle weakness and absent reflexes corresponding to nerve root level. A positive Spurling test is elicited where the patient's neck is extended and rotated whilst a downward pressure is applied to the head. Pain is noted to radiate down the ipsilateral limb towards the side to which the patient's head was rotated. Lhermitte's sign is negative in pure cervical radiculopathy (when the neck is flexed, the patient describes an electric shock sensation radiating down spine and into limbs, suggestive of cervical cord involvement).

Examination Findings for Cervical Radiculopathy

C5 radiculopathy	(Spondylosis, brachial neuritis) Weakness of biceps, spinati (infraspinatus, supraspinatus) and deltoid. Numbness over deltoid area. Absent biceps reflex.
C6 radiculopathy	(Spondylosis, disc herniation) Weakness of the biceps and brachioradialis muscles. Numbness over thumb and index finger. Absent supinator jerk.
C7 radiculopathy	(Disc herniation) Weakness of triceps muscle with numbness over middle finger. Absent triceps reflex.
C8–T1 radiculopathy	(Pancoast tumour, thoracic outlet syndrome) Weakness of small muscles of hand with atrophy. Numbness of little finger (C8).

Rotator Cuff Tears

Tears to the rotator cuff (supraspinatus, infraspinatus, subscapularis) are often due to chronic tendinitis (partial tears) or a sudden strain caused by a fall (complete tear). Partial tears present with a sustained painful arc in the absence of limitation of the range of movement, whilst complete tears restrict shoulder abduction to just 60° with a characteristic shrug when attempting to abduct beyond this. Full range of passive movements are present. When the arm is passively assisted above 90° of abduction, the patient is able to hold it in place and continue active abduction by utilising their deltoid muscles. However, on lowering their arm below 90° of abduction, the arm will suddenly drop (drop arm sign). Tenderness can be elicited under the acromion process. Partial and complete tears can be differentiated by infiltrating local anaesthetic into the shoulder joint, thereby eliminating pain and recovering full active abduction in a partial tear.

The Rotator Cuff Muscles

MNEMONIC: THE 'SITS' MUSCLES

Supraspinatus
Infraspinatus
Teres minor
Subscapularis

Frozen Shoulder (Adhesive Capsulitis)

Frozen shoulder (adhesive capsulitis) is a disorder characterised by pain, loss of motion and stiffness in the shoulder. The process involves thickening and contracture of the capsule surrounding the shoulder joint. It is more common in women between 40 and 60 years of age. In the elderly, it is normally preceded by a history of minor injury followed by progressively worsening pain in the shoulder that prevents the patient from sleeping on the affected side. The pain may subside after 9 months with stiffness intensifying and persisting over this time, limiting the range of movements of the shoulder. It is usually greater with internal rotation of the shoulder than with external rotation. Restriction of movement is often severe, with almost no glenohumeral movements possible. Stiffness begins to subside usually after 12 months with a return to full range of movement after 18 months.

Anterior Instability (Shoulder Dislocation)

Up to 95% of all shoulder dislocations occur anteriorly, commonly affecting men aged 18 to 25 years. This usually occurs when the arm is forced into abduction, external rotation and extension, i.e. when falling backward onto an outstretched hand. A patient with anterior dislocation presents holding the arm in slight abduction and internal rotation and reports pain with any attempt to rotate the arm. A mass may be palpable over the anterior shoulder. Occasionally, axillary nerve injury occurs with anterior dislocations manifesting as loss of sensation over the lateral deltoid as well as decreased strength of the deltoid muscle. Diagnosis is made by a positive apprehension test (see above).

6.3   ORTHOPAEDICS: ELBOW EXAMINATION

INSTRUCTIONS

Examine this patient who is complaining of pain in his elbow. Report your findings to the examiner as you go along, and make an appropriate diagnosis.

HISTORY

1 2 3

☐☐☐ **Introduction**   Introduce yourself. Elicit the patient's name, age and occupation. Establish rapport with the patient.

*History of Presenting Complaint

☐☐☐ **Pain**   'Where is the pain located? Does the pain move anywhere? What does the pain feel like? How severe is the pain, graded out of 10? What were you doing at the time it started?'

☐☐☐ **Stiffness**   'Do you have any stiffness in your elbow?'
       Swelling   'Have you noticed any swelling? Did it occur after an injury?'

☐☐☐ **Neurology**   'Have you noticed any tingling or numbness in your fingers? Do you have any weakness in your hands (ulnar nerve symptoms)?'

EXAMINATION

       Consent   Explain the examination to the patient and seek consent.

☐☐☐ **Expose**   Ask the patient to remove their upper garments in order to expose their elbows.

*Look

☐☐☐ **Inspect**   Inspect the elbows with the patient's arms by his sides. Look from the front, back and sides of the patient. Observe the skin, muscle and alignment.

Signs to Observe in the Elbow Examination

Skin	Scars, psoriatic plaques, rheumatoid nodules
Muscle	Wasting and fasciculation (biceps, triceps and brachioradialis)
Joints	Effusions (olecranon bursitis), gouty tophi
Alignment	Varus deformity (cubitus varus – supracondylar fracture)
	Valgus deformity (cubitus valgus – non-union of fractured lateral condyle)

*Feel

☐☐☐ **Palpate**   Ascertain if the elbow is painful. Ask the patient to locate the pain before palpating. Palpate the epicondyles and olecranon. Feel for any joint effusions or tenderness along the joint margin.

Signs to Palpate in the Elbow Examination

Skin	Temperature (infections, inflammation), subcutaneous nodules
Joints	Effusions, olecranon bursitis, synovial thickening, gouty tophi
Bones	Tenderness in the medial epicondyle (golfer's elbow) or lateral epicondyle (tennis elbow)

*Move

☐☐☐ **Movement**   Have the arms by the side of the patient. Assess the range of movement of the elbow during active and passive flexion (flexion deformity) and extension. Next check pronation (palms facing downwards) and supination (palms facing upwards) of the radioulnar joints with the elbows close to the patient's sides and flexed to 90°. Feel for crepitus during passive movements.

Difference between Supination and Pronation

Mnemonic:	**SUP**inated is the position of the forearm when carrying a bowl of **SOUP**
Mnemonic:	**PRO**nation is to turn your arm with the palm facing down as if you are **POUR**ing a jug of water

*Function

      Function   Ask the patient to put on a jacket or pour a glass of water.

☐☐☐ **Neurovascular**   State that you would like to check for the presence of any distal neurovascular deficits. Check for presence of a radial and brachial pulse. Also test sensation and proprioception in the hand, comparing both sides (ulnar nerve compression).

☐☐☐ **Summarise**   Thank the patient and offer to assist them to put on their clothes. Acknowledge the patient's concerns. Summarise your findings to the examiner.

'This is Mr Bob, a 35-year-old carpenter. He is right-handed, and has been complaining of pain in his right elbow which has been affecting his work. He recently started work on a building site fitting doors and noted the pain getting worse after this. On examination, both elbows appear normal with a full range of movements. However, on palpation there was significant tenderness over the right lateral epicondyle. The pain is reproduced on forced dorsiflexion of the wrist. In view of his history and examination, I believe that he suffers from tennis elbow.'

EXAMINER'S EVALUATION

1 2 3 4 5
☐☐☐☐☐ Overall assessment of elbow examination
☐☐☐☐☐ Role player's score
        Total mark out of 24

DIFFERENTIAL DIAGNOSIS

Elbow Deformities

Cubitus varus (Gunstock deformity) is a common complication of a supracondylar fracture. It describes an inward angulation of the distal segment of bone. The deformity is best seen with the elbow extended and arm elevated. Cubitus valgus is a common sequel of a disunited fractured lateral condyle. It is a deformity in which the elbow is turned out and a bony protrusion can be felt in the medial aspect of the joint. Possible complications include a delayed presentation of an ulnar nerve palsy which should be excluded.

Lateral Epicondylitis (Tennis Elbow)

Tennis elbow is an inflammatory condition of the wrist extensor tendons, particularly the extensor carpi radialis brevis, which attaches to the lateral epicondyle. It was termed 'tennis elbow' due to its association with athletes in racquet sports. However, most individuals who suffer from this condition sustain the injury at work, such as carpenters or house painters, by engaging in repetitive movements and unaccustomed strenuous activity involving the wrist. Peak incidence occurs between the ages of 30 and 50 years. Symptoms include pain of the lateral aspect of the elbow that is often severe and burning in nature and which gradually worsens over weeks or months. It is often aggravated by gripping, lifting or movements that involve extending the wrist such as pouring out a glass of water, turning a door handle or lifting a cup of coffee. On examination, tenderness is localised to the lateral epicondyle and can be reproduced by passively extending the wrist with the elbow held straight or when the patient resists forced dorsiflexion of the wrist.

Medial Epicondylitis (Golfer's Elbow)

Golfer's elbow, or medial epicondylitis, is similar to tennis elbow in presentation and pathology. It is due to inflammation of the wrist flexor tendon that attaches at the medial epicondyle. It is called 'golfer's elbow' due to its frequency in golfers, although individuals who have never played golf can develop the condition. The most common cause is overuse or repetitive stress of the flexor muscles involved in flexing the fingers and thumb, clenching the fist or supinating the wrist. These actions are often re-enacted as golfers take their swing but can also occur in other professions such as carpentry. On examination, tenderness is noted in the medial epicondyle which is reproducible when the patient resists forced flexion of the wrist.

Olecranon Bursitis

Olecranon bursitis is inflammation of the olecranon bursa as a result of direct trauma, prolonged pressure from leaning on a surface over a long duration, infection, or underlying medical conditions such as gout or rheumatoid arthritis. It presents as an impalpable small fluid-filled sac located at the tip of the elbow. It facilitates movement of the joint by permitting the skin to glide over the underlying bone. On examination, a tender, inflamed swelling is noted over the proximal end of the ulna. In the presence of infection, the overlying skin may become red and warm.

6.4   ORTHOPAEDICS: HAND EXAMINATION

INSTRUCTIONS

This patient has noticed pains in their hand. Examine the hand and report your findings to the examiner as you go along, and make an appropriate diagnosis.

HISTORY

1 2 3

☐☐☐ **Introduction**   Introduce yourself. Elicit the patient's name, age and occupation. Establish rapport with the patient.

*History of Presenting Complaint

History   'When did it first start, have you had this problem in the past, have you ever fallen, injured or fractured your hand before?'

☐☐☐ **Pain**   'Where is the pain located? Describe the nature of the pain. What makes it better or worse? Do you suffer from night pains?'

☐☐☐ **Stiffness**   'Do you suffer from stiffness in your joints? How long does it last for? Is it worse in the morning or the evening?'

Swelling   'Do you have any swelling in your joints?'

☐☐☐ **Sensation**   'Have you noticed any numbness or tingling in your hands?'

EXAMINATION

Consent   Obtain consent before beginning the examination.

☐☐☐ **Expose**   Ask the patient to expose their arms to above their elbows.

Pillow   Place a pillow on the patient's lap and ask them to rest their hands on it.

☐☐☐ **Pain**   Ask the patient before beginning the examination if they are in any pain. Do not shake the patient's hand as this might cause undue pain.

*Look

☐☐☐ **Inspect**   Examine both the dorsal and palmar surfaces of the hands and then examine them from the side with the patient's hands outstretched. Next inspect the hands in the praying position. Finally ask the patient to elevate their arms in the boxing position in order to inspect their elbows.

Signs to Observe in the Hand Examination

Hand	Nails	Nail fold infarcts, clubbing, psoriatic changes (pitting, onycholysis)
	Skin	Palmer erythema, Dupuytren's contracture, rheumatoid nodules
	Muscle	Wasting (1st dorsal interossei, thenar, hypothenar eminences)
	Joints	Swellings: Heberden's nodes (DIPJ) and Bouchard's nodes (PIPJ)
		Deformity: Swan neck, Boutonnière's deformity, z-shaped thumb
Wrists		Swelling, ganglion, vertical carpal scars
Elbows		Psoriatic plaques, gouty tophi, rheumatoid nodules

*Feel

☐☐☐ **Palpate**   Palpate the skin, assessing for temperature and joints for tenderness.

Skin   Run the back of your hand over the patient's forearm, hands and fingers to assess the temperature.

☐☐☐ *Joints*   Squeeze the patient's hands at the carpal and metacarpal joints and then each and every MCP and IP joint, assessing for tenderness and swelling of bone or soft tissue. Check for tenderness in the anatomical snuffbox (scaphoid fracture), the tip of the styloid process (de Quervain's disease) and the head of ulna (extensor carpi ulnaris tendinitis).

*Move

☐☐☐ **Movement**   Move each joint in the hand in turn noting any reduced movements.

Fingers   Hold each joint (MCP and IP) between your thumb and finger; flex and extend each joint in isolation. Assess for any limited range of movements. Ask the patient to make a precision grip by opposing their thumb to their index finger then attempt to break it with your index finger. Next, test grip strength by asking the patient to grab and squeeze your middle and index fingers. Compare grip strength on both sides.

☐☐☐ *Thumb*   Have the hands flat with the palms facing upwards. Test thumb abduction by asking the patient to point their thumbs to the ceiling and to hold it in position against the resistance of your finger. Test opposition by requesting the patient to make a ring with the tip of their little finger, maintaining it against resistance. Finally, ask the patient to place their thumb firmly against their palm for adduction and to stretch out their thumb to the opposite side for extension.

☐☐☐ *Wrist*   Ask the patient to perform wrist flexion (80°) and wrist dorsiflexion (80°). If possible, test for radial (40°) and ulnar deviation (10°) as well as pronation and supination.

Nerve Supply to Muscles in the Hand

MNEMONIC: 'LOAF'

Median nerve (ape hand) — Lateral two **L**umbricals, **O**pponens pollicis, **A**bductor pollicis brevis, **F**lexor pollicis brevis

MNEMONIC: 'BESTS'

Radial nerve (wrist drop) — **B**rachioradialis, **E**xtensors of wrist, **S**upinator, **T**riceps, loss of **S**ensation over the anatomical snuffbox

MNEMONIC: 'MAFIA'

Ulnar nerve (claw hand) — **M**edial lumbricals, **A**dductor pollicis (pincer grip), **F**irst dorsal interossei, **I**nterossei, **A**bductor digiti minimi

*Sensation

☐☐☐ **Neurology** — Assess sensation in the hand by testing light touch. Touch a wisp of cotton over the little finger (ulnar nerve), index finger (median nerve) and the lateral aspect of the thumb or anatomical snuff box (radial nerve). Ask permission to formally assess pain sensation using a neurological pin. Test both sides and compare.

*Function

☐☐☐ **Daily Tasks** — Assess function by asking the patient to carry out everyday tasks such as undoing buttons and writing a sentence using a pen or holding a cup.

*Special Tests

☐☐☐ **Tinel's Sign** — Tap over the median nerve (carpal tunnel) at the wrist to reproduce symptoms of pain or tingling in the distribution of the median nerve.

Tinel's sign

Tap over the median nerve at the wrist to reproduce symptoms in the fingers and thumb.

□□□   **Phalen's Test**   Hold the wrists fully hyperflexed for 1–2 minutes to reproduce symptoms of pain or tingling in the distribution of the median nerve.

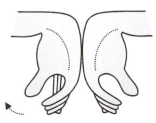

Phalen's test

Have the wrists fully hyperflexed for one minute to reproduce symptoms in the fingers and thumb.

□□□   **Fromen's Sign**   Ask the patient to clutch a piece of paper between their thumb and index finger. Attempt to pull the paper away from the clasp of the patient. If the thumb adductor is weak then the patient can only hold onto the paper by flexing the interphalangeal joints of the thumb and is unable to hold the thumb straight (ulnar nerve compression).

□□□   **Flexor Digitorum Profundus**

Ask the patient to flex the distal interphalangeal joint while holding the finger in extension at the proximal interphalangeal joint.

□□□   **Flexor Digitorum Superficialis**

Hold all the fingers in full extension except for the finger being tested. Ask the patient to flex the remaining finger at the proximal interphalangeal joint.

Anatomy of the Flexor Digitorum Muscles

Mnemonic: 'Superficialis splits in two, to permit profundus passing through.'

□□□   **Summarise**   Thank the patient. Acknowledge the patient's concerns. Restore the patient's clothing. Summarise your findings to the examiner.

'This is Mrs Susan Gregory, a 40-year-old pregnant woman. She is complaining of hand pains that are worse during the night. She has to shake her hands in order to relieve the pain. The pain is described as a burning sensation. On examination, the patient has pain and burning in the median nerve distribution. Her power and joint movements were normal. However, Tinel's and Phalen's test were positive. From the history and examination findings, I believe that this patient has carpal tunnel syndrome. I would like to perform a nerve conduction test to confirm my suspicions.'

EXAMINER'S EVALUATION

DIFFERENTIAL DIAGNOSIS

Carpal Tunnel Syndrome

Carpal tunnel syndrome is caused by the entrapment of the median nerve in the carpal tunnel due to pressure. It usually affects patients between 40 and 50 years of age and is eight times more frequent in women than in men. It can be due to hypothyroidism, diabetes mellitus, pregnancy, obesity, rheumatoid arthritis and acromegaly; however, in most cases the cause is unknown. Symptoms include burning pain and tingling felt in the distribution of the median nerve (thumb, index, middle and lateral half of the ring finger). The pain is usually worse at night but can be relieved by shaking the wrist. On examination there is loss of sensation in the median nerve distribution, wasting of the thenar eminence and weakness of the abductor pollicis brevis. The diagnosis can be confirmed with a positive Phalen's and Tinel's test.

Treatment of Carpal Tunnel Syndrome

MNEMONIC: 'WRIST'

Wear splints at night, **R**est, **I**nject steroid, **S**urgical decompression, **T**ake diuretics

---

Trigger Finger (Stenosing Tenosynovitis)

The flexor tendons extend from the wrist to the fingers. Occasionally a flexor tendon may become trapped in the opening of its sheath due to nodules or a thickening of the tendon sheath. Trigger finger can affect any finger, but the middle and ring fingers are most commonly affected. Patients note a clicking noise when the finger is flexed with the affected finger remaining bent when the others are extended. With some effort the tendon can be suddenly freed ('triggering') and the finger snaps back into place.

Mallet's Finger

Mallet's finger, otherwise known as 'baseball finger', is a deformity of the finger where the distal interphalangeal joint is held in the flexed position. It is a common sports injury and occurs when a ball strikes the tip of the finger or thumb causing either rupture to the extensor tendon or an avulsion fracture. As a result the patient is unable to extend and straighten the distal joint of the finger.

De Quervain's Disease (Stenosing Tenosynovitis)

Repetitive abduction and adduction of the thumb can irritate the tendons of the extensor pollicis brevis and abductor pollicis longus muscles, which can become inflamed and thickened. This can occur from repetitive actions which require much force, such as pruning a hedge.

When this occurs, any movement of the thumb (in particular, gripping) may cause pain at the radial side of the wrist. On examination, there may be swelling overlying the tendons of the thumb. Tenderness can be located at the tip of the radial styloid where the tendons of the extensor pollicis brevis and longus cross. Passive stretching of the tendons as well as abduction of the thumb against resistance and passive adduction are extremely painful. The diagnosis can be confirmed with a positive Eichoff's test. Eichoff's test consists of flexing the thumb across the palm inside a clenched fist and placing the wrist in ulnar deviation. This stretches the inflamed tendons over the radial styloid, reproducing the patient's pain.

Eichoff's Test

Clench the thumb inside a closed fist and tilt the hand into forward flexion. Note a sharp pain over the radial styloid suggesting De Quervain's tenosynovitis.

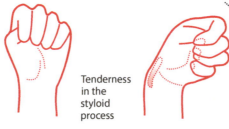

Tenderness in the styloid process

Forward flexion of the wrist generates pain

6.5   ORTHOPAEDICS: HIP EXAMINATION

INSTRUCTIONS

Please examine this patient, who is complaining of pain and stiffness in the hip. Report your findings to the examiner as you go along, and make an appropriate diagnosis.

HISTORY

1 2 3

☐☐☐   **Introduction**   Introduce yourself. Elicit the patient's name, age and occupation. Establish rapport with the patient.

*History of Presenting Complaint

History   'When did it first start? Have you had this problem in the past? Have you ever fallen, injured or fractured your hip before?'

☐☐☐   **Pain**   'Where is the pain located? Does the pain move anywhere? How severe is the pain, graded out of 10? What does the pain feel like?'

Pain in the hip may be felt in the groin or inner thigh. It often radiates to the knee. Hip pain is often made worse by exercise or walking.

Stiffness   'Do you have any stiffness in your hip? Is it worse in the morning or evening? Does it come on suddenly or gradually?'

General Health   'How is your general health? Do you have any malaise, fever or weight loss?'

☐☐☐   **Impact on Life**   'How has your hip problem affected your daily activities and/or mobility?'

EXAMINATION

Consent   Obtain consent before beginning the examination.

☐☐☐   **Expose**   Ask the patient if they can undress to their undergarments.

*Look

☐☐☐   **General**   With the patient standing, look for alignment of the shoulders, hips and patella and ensure that the ASISs (anterior superior iliac spine) are aligned and at the same level to one other. Inspect from behind for scoliosis and gluteal wasting. Inspect from the side for increased lumbar lordosis (fixed flexion deformity).

☐☐☐   **Gait**   Observe their gait. Ask the patient if they can walk to the end of the room and return.

Signs to Look for in Gait

Use of a walking aid	Sticks, frames
Speed	Rhythm, presence of a limp
Phases of walking	Heel strike, stance, push off and swing
Stride length	Reduced, limited
Arm swing	Present, absent
Types of gait	Such as Trendelenburg's and antalgic gait
Trendelenburg's gait	Ineffective hip abduction results in the pelvis dropping during the weight-bearing stance phase and the body leaning to the unaffected side
Antalgic gait	Pain in the hip causing a shortening of the stance phase and the body leaning to the affected side. Most common cause is osteoarthritis

☐☐☐   **Trendelenburg**   The Trendelenburg test is used to assess hip stability. Instruct the patient to stand upon the sound limb while raising the opposite foot by bending it at the knee. Carefully observe, or palpate with a hand on the iliac crest, for pelvic tilting and noting which side it drops towards. Repeat the test but on the opposite leg.

Interpreting Trendelenburg's Test

Negative test	Pelvis rises on the opposite, unsupported side
Positive test	Pelvis drops on the opposite, unsupported side
Causes	Dislocation of the hip, weakness of the abductor muscles, shortening of femoral neck, pain in the hip

In general, when standing on one leg the weight-bearing hip is held stable by the abductor muscles, which contract, elevating the pelvis on the unsupported side. However, if the hip is unstable, abduction of the hip does not occur and the pelvis drops on the unsupported side.

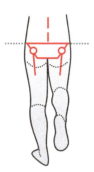
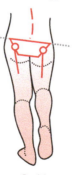

Negative
Trendelenburg's
test (normal)

Positive
Trendelenburg's
test (abnormal)

Trendelenburg's test

Ask the patient to stand on one leg while flexing the opposite leg at the knee keeping their foot off the ground. Normally, the hip is held stable by the abductor muscles contracting in the supporting leg. A positive Trendelenburg's sign is noted if the pelvis drops on the unsupported side.

☐☐☐ **Observe**   Inspect the hip with the patient lying on the couch.

Signs to Look for in the Hip Examination

Skin	Scars, sinus, pigmentation, unusual skin creases	
Muscle	Wasting, fasciculations	
Swelling	Look for effusion in hip or knee (effusions in knee joint – OA)	
Position	*Shortened limb*	Ankle misalignment with pelvic tilting
	Limb rotation	Externally (#NOF, femoral shaft) or internally
	Fixed flexion deformity	Excessive lordosis

☐☐☐ **Measure**   Before measuring the length of the limbs, square the pelvis by ensuring that the iliac crests are aligned and on the same level. Inability to square the pelvis indicates possible fixed adduction or abduction deformity of the hip.

Measure the apparent limb length by measuring the distance from the xiphisternum to the medial malleolus on each side. Then measure the distance between the ASIS to the medial malleolus on each side to assess the true limb length. Compare the two values.

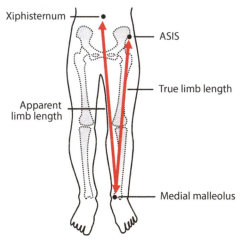

Xiphisternum

ASIS

True limb length

Apparent limb length

Medial malleolus

Apparent and true limb length

Measure the distance from the xiphisternum to the medial malleolus for the apparent limb length. Measure the distance from the ASIS to the medial malleolus for the true limb length.

If the apparent limb lengths appear unequal but with no disparity between the true limb lengths, this could be due to a fixed adduction deformity of the hip. If the true limb length measurements appear unequal then there is true limb shortening.

Causes of Limb Length Inequality

True shortening	Perthes' disease, slipped femoral epiphysis, avascular necrosis, arthritis, hip dislocation
Apparent shortening	Fixed adduction deformity of hip (arthritis)

*Feel

☐☐☐   **Palpate**   Palpate the hip with the patient still lying on the couch. Feel the hip for temperature, effusions and bony landmarks.

Signs to Palpate in the Hip Examination

Skin	Temperature (infections, inflammation), soft tissue contours
Joints	Effusion in the hip
Bones	Palpate for tenderness over the greater trochanter (bursitis), lesser trochanter (tears of the iliopsoas), ischial tuberosity (tears of the hamstrings), feel for bony landmarks – (greater trochanter, ASIS)

*Move

Note any limited range of movements or the reporting of pain. Examine each joint actively first by asking the patient to perform the movement independently. Re-examine the joint passively by helping the patient move the joint.

☐☐☐   **Flexion**   Have the patient flex their knees and move their hip joint into the flexed position as far as possible (normal range 130°).

☐☐☐   **Thomas' Test**   Keep one hand flat on the examining table under the patient's lumbar spine. Have both hips flexed then ask the patient to hold on to his sound knee (sound hip is flexed to limit) while straightening the suspect leg. If the limb is elevated off the examining table and is unable to fully straighten then there is a fixed flexion deformity of the hip on the affected side. The angle through which the thigh is raised from the couch is the angle of fixed flexion. Repeat the test for the other hip.

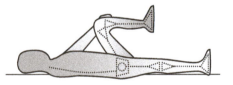

Normal

The patient lies flat on his back while holding one of his legs and completely straightens the other. The test is normal if the limb is not elevated off the couch.

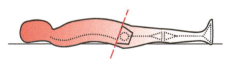

Fixed flexion deformity

Patient arches the spine and pelvis to compensate for a fixed flexion deformity of the hip. An exaggerated lumbar lordosis is noted.

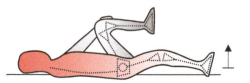

Positive Thomas' Test

Flexion of the hip and knee exposes a fixed flexion deformity on the affected side with the limb unable to be fully straightened and raised off the couch.

□□□ *Rotation* — Have the hip and knee flexed at 90°. Hold the knee with one hand and the ankle with the other. Now move the foot medially for external rotation (45°) of the hip, and laterally for internal rotation (45°).

□□□ *Abduction* — Drop one leg over the side of couch. Place one hand on the ASIS to fix the pelvis and the other on the available ankle. Abduct the leg through its full range of movement (45°). Repeat for the other leg.

□□□ *Adduction* — Have both legs restored on the bed and adduct one leg by crossing it over the other (30°). Repeat for the other leg.

□□□ **Neurovascular** — State that you would like to check for the presence of any distal neurovascular deficits. Check for presence of peripheral pulses (dorsalis pedis and posterior tibial arteries). Also test sensation and proprioception along the leg comparing both sides.

Age of Incidence of Common Hip Disorders

Incidence	Hip condition
0–2 years	Developmental dislocation of the hip (DDH)
2–5 years	TB arthritis, pyogenic arthritis, irritable hip syndrome
5–10 years	Perthes' disease, irritable hip syndrome
10–20 years	Slipped upper femoral epiphysis
20–50 years	Osteoarthritis (secondary)
50–100 years	Osteoarthritis (primary), rheumatoid arthritis

□□□ **Summarise** — Thank the patient and offer to assist them to put on their clothes. Acknowledge the patient's concerns. Summarise your findings to the examiner.

'This is Mrs Smith, a 60-year-old widow who has been complaining of hip pain for a number of years. She states the pain is getting worse, particularly at end of the day and during periods of activity. The pain radiates to her thigh and is not controlled by her usual analgesia. On examination, there is an antalgic gait with a positive Trendelenburg's test, reduced generalised movement of the hip and a positive Thomas' test. In view of these findings, I believe that Mrs Smith suffers from osteoarthritis. However, I would like to perform an X-ray to exclude other causes (rheumatoid arthritis, neck of femur fracture).'

EXAMINER'S EVALUATION

1 2 3 4 5
□□□□□ Overall assessment of hip examination
□□□□□ Role player's score
Total mark out of 33

DIFFERENTIAL DIAGNOSIS

Osteoarthritis of the Hip

Osteoarthritis in the hip can be primary in nature or secondary to Perthes' diseases (in the young), rheumatoid arthritis and Paget's (in the elderly). Symptoms include pain and stiffness in the hip. Symptoms progress slowly over time (years) with pain precipitated by lesser activity (shorter distances walked) as the disease worsens. Osteoarthritis tends to occur in patients over the age of 50 since the risk of wear and tear on the joint increases with age. The pain originates in the groin and may radiate to the knee. Pain usually occurs after a period of activity while stiffness occurs after periods of rest. On examination, the patient may reveal a positive Trendelenburg's sign with a limp in the gait. The affected leg is held externally rotated and in adduction appearing short in limb length, whilst the Thomas' test may expose the presence of a fixed flexion deformity. There is also a general restriction in limb movements.
X-ray demonstrating OA of the right hip typified by the loss of joint space.

Slipped Femoral Epiphysis

Slipped upper femoral epiphysis is a disease of adolescence where the upper femoral epiphysis slips downwards from its normal position on the femoral neck, causing a coxa vara deformity. It is a common cause of hip and knee pain in those aged between 10 and 20 and is the most common hip disorder in adolescence. It is three times more common in boys than it is in girls and commonly affects the left hip more than the right, though bilateral slips do occur. The condition is linked with overweight (obesity) from endocrine disorders (hypothyroidism, hypopituitarism, growth hormone deficiency) and occasionally there is a history of preceding trauma. The patient may complain of pain in the hip or knee and walks with a limp. In the acute setting weight bearing is impossible. On examination, there is a loss of motion in the hip joint, particularly internal rotation, and abduction of the affected hip. Forceful examination of the restricted movements will exacerbate the pain. The limb is externally rotated with true shortening of the leg causing an inequality in limb length.

Trochanteric Bursitis

The trochanteric bursa is found overlying the greater trochanter of the femur. Inflammation can occur from either acute trauma, such as a fall or a football tackle, or more commonly from repetitive, cumulative trauma. Classically, there is pain over the greater trochanteric region of the lateral hip. The pain is made worse when the patient lies on the affected bursa and can awaken the patient at night. Symptoms tend to get worse with walking. On examination, the range of motion is generally preserved. Tenderness can be elicited on direct palpation over the bursa.

6.6   ORTHOPAEDICS: KNEE EXAMINATION

INSTRUCTIONS

Please examine this patient who is complaining of pain and stiffness in the knee. Report your findings to the examiner as you go along, and make an appropriate diagnosis.

HISTORY

1 2 3

☐☐☐   **Introduction**   Introduce yourself. Elicit the patient's name, age and occupation. Establish rapport with the patient.

*History of Presenting Complaint

History   'When did it first start? Have you had this problem in the past? Have you ever fallen, injured or fractured your knee before?'

☐☐☐   **Pain**   'Where is the pain located? Does the pain move anywhere? How severe is the pain, graded out of 10? What does the pain feel like?'

☐☐☐   **Stiffness**   'Do you have any stiffness? Is it worse in the morning or the evening?'

Swelling   'Have you noticed any swelling? Did it occur after an injury? How long after did it occur (immediately – haemarthrosis; some hours after – torn meniscus)?'

☐☐☐   **Locking**   'Have you noticed that you are unable to fully straighten your leg when you walk (torn meniscus)?'

☐☐☐   **Giving Way**   'Have you ever felt that your knee was about to give way (torn meniscus, torn ligament, patella dislocation)?'

☐☐☐   **Impact on Life**   'How has your knee problem affected your daily activities and/or mobility?'

EXAMINATION

Consent   Obtain consent before beginning the examination.

☐☐☐   **Expose**   Ask the patient if they can undress to their undergarments.

*Look

Gait   Assess the patient's gait by asking the patient if they could walk to the end of the room and return. Observe the phases of gait, the presence of a limp and for restriction of movement.

☐☐☐   **General**   Inspect the patient standing, then lying on the couch in the supine position. Look at the posture, position and alignment of the knees. Measure the quadriceps girth 10 cm above the patella for wasting on both legs.

Signs to Look for in the Knee Examination

Observe with the patient standing	
Posture	Alignment of shoulder, hips and patella
Joint	Inspect the popliteal fossa from the back for a Baker's cyst
Position	Neutral, valgus (knock knee), varus (bow leg) deformity,
	Fixed flexion deformity/attitude, recurvatum (hyperextension)
Observe with the patient lying on the couch	
Skin	Colour, sinuses, scars (arthroscopic)
Muscle	Wasting (quadriceps – vastus medialis), fasciculations
Joints	Effusions, rheumatoid arthritis nodules, psoriatic plaques
Alignment	Patellar alignment, tibial alignment
Position	Fixed flexion deformity of the knee (unable to straighten the knee)

*Feel

☐☐☐ **General**   Palpate the knee with the patient still lying on the couch. Before palpating it, ask if there is any pain. Feel the knee for warmth, effusions and position. State that you would like to perform the patella apprehension test to test for patella dislocation.

Skin   Feel over the knee for warmth and temperature (infections, inflammation) comparing both knees.

☐☐☐ **Effusions**   Perform the cross-fluctuation, patella tap test and bulge test to assess the size of the effusion.

Cross-fluctuat.   One hand empties the suprapatellar pouch while the other hand is placed just below the patella. A positive test is seen when an impulse is transmitted across the joint with alternate compressions. This test is used to detect large effusions.

Patella Tap   Empty the suprapatellar pouch with one hand and then sharply tap the patella with the index finger.

A positive patella tap test will see the patella sink, striking the femur then bouncing back up again. This test elicits moderately sized effusions.

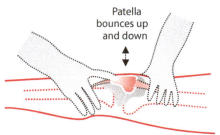

Patella bounces up and down

Patella Tap Test

Slide your hand down the patient's thigh emptying the suprapatellar pouch forcing the effusion below the patella. Next sharply tap the patella with the index finger of the other hand. Note if the patella bounces up.

Bulge Test   After draining the medial compartment by massaging the medial aspect of the joint, swiftly stroke the lateral aspect of the knee, and observe for the appearance of a ripple on the medial surface. This test can detect the presence of small effusions in the joint.

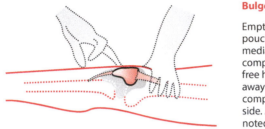

Bulge Test

Empty the suprapatellar pouch before emptying the medial compartment by compressing it with your free hand. Lift the hand away and then quickly compress the lateral side. A positive test is noted if a 'bulge' is seen on the medial surface.

☐☐☐ **Joints**

Have the knee flexed at 90° and feel along the joint line for tenderness. Feel for the ligaments and synovial thickening, as well as bony landmarks such as the tibial tuberosity and femoral condyles. Palpate in the popliteal fossa for a Baker's cyst.

Patella

Ask permission to perform the patella apprehension test. Flex the knee while pressing the patella laterally.

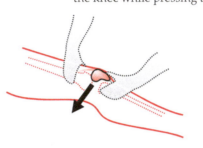

Patella Apprehension Test

Flex the knee to approximately 30 degrees while pushing the patella firmly in the lateral direction. The patient will anticipate patella dislocation and discontinue the test.

If the patella is unstable, the patient will anticipate patella dislocation and discontinue the test.

*Move

☐☐☐ **Active**

Note any limited range of movement or the reporting of pain. Test for knee flexion by asking the patient to bend their leg backwards without providing assistance. Then ask them to straighten their leg as far as possible for knee extension.

Passive

Place one hand on the knee and the other on the ankle. Attempt to flex the patient's knee back as far as possible (140°). Then test for extension by straightening the leg while feeling for crepitus in the knee (–10°).

*Special Tests

☐☐☐ **Collateral Lig.**

The medial and lateral collateral ligaments can be assessed by applying a valgus or varus force at the knee. Have the patient's foot tucked under your armpit while holding the patient's knee with both hands. Apply a valgus force by steering the knee medially to test the medial ligament. Next apply a varus stress by pushing the knee laterally to test for the lateral ligament. Alternatively, hold the ankle in one hand and the knee in the other. Test the medial ligament by abducting the ankle whilst pushing the knee medially. Test the lateral ligament by adducting the ankle whilst pushing the knee laterally. Apply the stresses at 0° and repeat with the leg slightly flexed at 20°. Excessive movement suggests a torn or stretched collateral ligament.

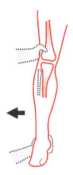

Test medial collaterals

Hold the patient's ankle in one hand and the knee in the other. Test for medial instability by applying a valgus stress to the knee while abducting the ankle.

Excessive joint movement

Test lateral collaterals

Hold the patient's ankle in one hand and the knee in the other. Test for lateral instability by applying a varus stress to the knee while adducting the ankle.

Excessive joint movement

Cruciate Lig.   Look for the sag sign and perform the Drawer test and Lachman test to assess the cruciate ligaments.

Sag Sign   Have the knee flexed to 90° and observe for sagging of the upper end of the tibia compared to the patella. The sag sign indicates a posterior cruciate ligament tear.

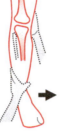

Sag Sign

Observe for the posterior tibial sag sign by having the patient's knee in 90 degrees of flexion. Note the sagging of the tibia suggesting the presence of a posterior cruciate ligament tear. Compare the knee to the opposite side.

☐☐☐ *Drawer Test*   Ask the patient if they have any pain in their feet.
Have the knee flexed to 90° and then anchor the foot by sitting on it, requesting permission before doing so. Hold the knee with your thumbs on the tibial tuberosity and fingers in the popliteal fossa; rock it back and forth assessing for any give. An excessive anterior movement indicates anterior cruciate laxity while an excessive posterior movement suggest posterior cruciate laxity.

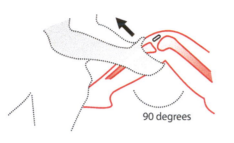

Drawer Test

Have the patient's knee flexed to 90 degrees before sitting on his foot. Grasp hold of the proximal tibia with both hands with thumbs on the tibial tuberosity and fingers in the popliteal fossa. Pull the tibia forward while noting degree of anterior tibial displacement.

90 degrees

Lachman Test

Have the patient's knee flexed to 20°. Hold the lower thigh in one hand and place the other hand behind the proximal tibia. Gently glide the tibia forward by pulling anteriorly. An intact anterior cruciate should prevent the forward gliding movement of the tibia on the femur. The Lachman test is a more sensitive test for anterior cruciate ligament laxity and is often carried out if the Drawer test cannot be performed due to foot pain, for example.

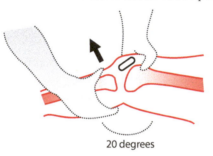

Lachman Test

Have the patient's knee flexed at 20 degrees. Stabilise the femur with one hand and place the other hand behind the proximal tibia with the thumb on the tibial tuberosity. Attempt to pull the tibia anteriorly checking for forward translational movement.

20 degrees

Meniscus Tears

Perform the McMurray test and Apley's grinding test to assess for torn meniscal tags.

☐☐☐ *McMurray Test*

Before undertaking this test, warn the patient that this test may cause pain. Flex the knee as far as possible while holding the knee joint. Externally rotate the leg and slowly extend it while stressing it into valgus. Repeat, but this time internally rotate

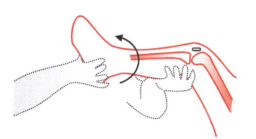

McMurray Test

Flex the patient's knee and have one hand stablising the knee with the other hand holding the sole of the foot. Test for a medial meniscus tag by externally rotating the leg and applying a valgus stress while slowly extending the knee. Test for lateral meniscal tags by repeating the test but internally rotating the knee while applying a varus stress.

Externally rotate the leg and extend while applying a valgus stress.

the leg and extend it while stressing it into varus. A positive test is signalled by a painful click felt or heard. This indicates that a torn meniscal tag is caught between the articular surfaces of the femoral condyle and the tibial plateau.

Grinding Test   Ask permission to perform Apley's grinding test. Have the patient lying prone with their knee flexed to 90° and rest your knee on the patient's thigh. Apply a grinding force by rotating and applying compression to the knee joint. Elicited pain suggests a torn meniscus. Repeat but instead rotate and pull the leg upwards simultaneously with patient's thigh anchored down with your knee. Pain indicates ligament damage.

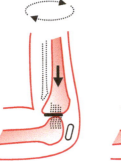 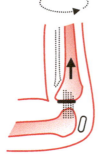

Apley's Grinding Test

Test for a meniscal tear by applying pressure and rotational force to the foot with the patient lying prone with his knee flexed 90 degrees. Test for ligament damage by reversing the direction of pressure and rotation. Elicit pain for a positive test.

☐☐☐ **Neurovascular**   State that you would like to check for the presence of any distal neurovascular deficits. Check for presence of peripheral pulses (dorsalis pedis and posterior tibial arteries). Also test sensation and proprioception along both legs comparing both sides.

Request   State that you would also like to perform a hip and ankle examination.

☐☐☐ **Summarise**   Thank the patient and offer to assist them to put on their clothes. Acknowledge the patient's concerns and encourage questions. Summarise your findings to the examiner.

'This is Mark Hughes, a 20-year-old man who was playing football on the weekend. He is complaining of sharp pain in the medial aspect of the knee. He states that when he was playing football he twisted his knee. Shortly afterward he developed pain and swelling. Now he notes that his knee does not fully extend and can occasionally give way. On examination, he has a large fluctuant bulge on the medial aspect of the knee, and walks with an antalgic gait. The swelling had a positive bulge test. Of note is that he also had a positive McMurray test. In view of his history and examination findings I suspect he has a meniscal tear.'

EXAMINER'S EVALUATION

DIFFERENTIAL DIAGNOSIS

Osteoarthritis of the Knee

The knee represents the commonest site of presentation for osteoarthritis. It can be primary in nature or secondary due to injury, torn meniscus, recurrent patella dislocation or ligament instability. Patients are classically over 50 years of age, overweight and may have a bow-leg deformity. They often complain of pain with stiffness. The pain originates in the knee and is severe in nature. It is made worse after the individual attempts to move after a period of inactivity. However, stiffness usually occurs after periods of rest. On examination, there may be limited movement with patellofemoral crepitus and flexion or varus deformities. The quadriceps muscle is often wasted and there is no effusion or warmth.

   X-rays will typically demonstrate loss of joint space, osteophytes, subchondral sclerosis and subchondral cysts.

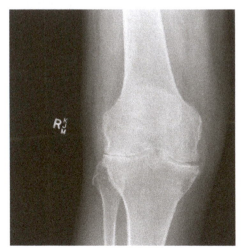

Meniscal Tears

The menisci are C-shaped cartilaginous tissues that are located above, and in addition to, the articular cartilage of the tibia. They act as shock absorbers and provide smooth movement and stability in the knee joint. Meniscal tears are common sport injuries in young athletes. They result from a twisting force applied to a bent knee that is also weight-bearing, commonly seen in footballers as they strike a ball or when they are running and attempt to change direction. Tears vary in size and location and can be partial or full length. Longitudinal tears that extend along the length of the meniscus, with the cartilage still attached front and back, are known as a bucket handle tear. The 'handle' may flip over, displace and be caught between the femur and tibia, locking the knee and preventing full extension. Symptoms of meniscal tears include pain, swelling and loss of knee function. The pain often occurs when attempting to extend the leg and is felt within the knee joint. Swelling of the knee often develops several hours after the injury as a result of inflammation caused by the tear. The patient may describe that his knee occasionally gives way with pain and swelling developing afterwards. The locking of the knee is synonymous with bucket handle tears. Often patients are able to manually manipulate their leg and 'unlock' the knee so that it can be straightened once again. On examination, the knee is held partially flexed, there is localised tenderness in the joint line, an effusion is often present and there is limitation to knee extension. McMurray and Apley's grinding tests are positive.

Baker's Cyst

Baker's cyst is a collection of fluid in the synovial sac which protrudes out of the back of the knee below the joint line from the popliteal fossa. It is differentiated from a popliteal aneurysm by the absence of a palpable pulse. This type of Baker's cyst is commonly associated with a tear in the meniscal cartilage of the knee. In older adults, this condition is frequently associated with degenerative arthritis of the knee. It can present as a painless or painful swelling behind the knee. Occasionally, the cyst may rupture, causing pain, swelling and bruising on the back of the knee and calf. Transillumination of the cyst can demonstrate that the mass is fluid-filled.

Bursitis

The semimembranosus bursa (Brodie's bursa) is found between the medial head of gastroc-nemius and the semimembranosus tendon. Inflammation of the bursa presents as a painless fluctuant lump within the medial aspect of the popliteal fossa behind the knee. It is best examined whilst standing with the knee in extension. Prepatellar bursitis (housemaid's knee) is caused by repeated friction between the skin and the patella. It used to be synonymous with housemaids due to the time they spent washing floors on their knees. However, it now occurs more often in carpet fitters and miners. On examination, a swelling can be noted directly over the patella. The rest of the knee examination is unremarkable. Infrapatellar bursitis (clergy-man's knees) similarly is caused by friction between the skin and patella. However, the swelling is found distal to the patella and superficial to the patellar ligament. This is caused by the kneeling posture taken up by a person in prayer as opposed to the one who cleans floors.

6.7   ORTHOPAEDICS: ANKLE AND FOOT EXAMINATION

INSTRUCTIONS

Examine this patient, who is complaining of sudden onset of ankle pain. Report your findings to the examiner as you go along, and make an appropriate diagnosis.

HISTORY

1 2 3
☐☐☐ **Introduction**   Introduce yourself. Elicit the patient's name, age and occupation. Establish rapport with the patient.

*History of Presenting Complaint

☐☐☐ **Pain**   'Where is the pain located? Does the pain move anywhere? How severe is the pain graded out of 10? Can you describe the pain? What were you doing at the time it first started?'

☐☐☐ **Stiffness**   'Do you have any stiffness in your ankle or foot?'
Swelling   'Have you noticed any swelling (bunion, gout)?'

EXAMINATION

Consent   Explain the examination to the patient and seek consent.
☐☐☐ **Expose**   Ask the patient to expose his lower limbs including his feet.

*Gait

☐☐☐ **Walk**   Observe the patient's gait. Ask the patient if they could walk to the end of the room and return. Note the presence of an antalgic gait.

Signs to Look for in Gait

Use of a walking aid	Sticks, frames
Speed	Rhythm, presence of a limp
Phases of walking	Heel strike, stance, push off and swing
Stride length	Reduced, limited
Arm swing	Present, absent

*Look

☐☐☐ **Inspect**   Look at the patient's shoes for signs of abnormal wear.
Inspect with the patient standing and then observe the ankles and feet from behind. Assess the patient's posture, alignment of the feet and joint deformity.
Ask the patient to lie down on the couch and continue your inspection.

Signs to Look for in the Ankle and Foot Examination

Skin	Colour, scars, sinus, corns, callosities, ulcers, fungal infections, in-growing toenails
Muscle	Wasting of the calf (gastrocnemius) and lower leg muscles
Alignment	Valgus deformity (foot deviated away from the midline)
	Varus deformity (foot deviated to the midline)
Deformity	Pes planus (flat foot), pes cavus (high-arched foot), talipes (club foot)
	Bunion (1st MTP joint), hallux valgus/rigidus, claw toe, mallet toe, hammer toe

*Feel

☐☐☐ **Palpate**   Ascertain if the foot is painful. Ask the patient to locate the pain before palpating it. Assess the skin temperature by running the back of your hands along both feet simultaneously comparing both sides. Palpate for presence of peripheral pulses. Palpate the joint margin, hindfoot, midfoot and forefoot noting any tenderness.

Signs to Palpate in the Ankle and Foot Examination

Skin	Temperature (infections, inflammation)
Pulses	Dorsalis pedis, posterior tibial
Joints	Effusions, oedema, lumps
Bones	Localise any tenderness (malleoli, MTP, IP, metatarsal head)

*Move

☐☐☐ **Movement**   Assess the range of movement at the ankle, subtalar, midtarsal joints and toes. Check active and passive movements for each joint.

Ankle   Grasp the heel in one hand and hold the midfoot in the other. Test ankle dorsiflexion (10°) and plantar-flexion (40°).

Subtalar   Maintain your grasp of the patient's foot. Using the ankle as a pivot, assess foot inversion (30°) by directing the sole towards the midline and foot eversion (30°) by turning the sole away from the midline.

Midtarsal   Hold the heel firmly in one hand and the forefoot in the other to stabilise the subtalar joint. Attempt to move the forefoot up and down and then from side to side.

Toe   Assess flexion and extension in each toe in turn.

*Special Tests

☐☐☐ **Simmonds' Test**   Before performing this test, palpate the calf muscle and Achilles tendon for wasting and tenderness. Note for depression in the lower calf signifying a tendon rupture. Perform Simmonds' test to confirm a ruptured Achilles tendon. Have the patient lying prone with their feet hanging off the edge of the bed. Squeeze the calves simultaneously and note for reflex plantarflexion in both feet. Absence of plantarflexion of a foot suggests a ruptured tendon.

Simmonds' Test

Examine the patient lying flat on the couch with legs hanging off the edge. Squeeze both calves simultaneously and note plantarflexion in both feet. Absence of plantarflexion in a foot is a positive test and suggestive of a ruptured Achilles tendon.

☐☐☐ **Neurovascular** — State that you would like to check for the presence of any distal neurovascular deficits. Perform a full arterial examination to check for the presence of peripheral pulses. Test sensation and proprioception along both legs and feet, comparing both sides.

Request — State that you would also like to perform a hip and knee examination.

☐☐☐ **Summarise** — Thank the patient and offer to assist them to put on their clothes. Acknowledge the patient's concerns. Summarise your findings to the examiner.

'Mr Peckham, a 15-year-old teenager, complains of sudden onset of pain in his right lower ankle. On examination, he was found to walk with an antalgic gait and unable to bear weight fully on his right side. A depression was noted in his right lower calf, with weakness of plantar flexion of the ankle. Simmonds' test was positive. In view of the history and examination, I suspect Mr Peckham has a ruptured right Achilles tendon.'

EXAMINER'S EVALUATION

1 2 3 4 5
☐☐☐☐☐ Overall assessment of ankle and foot examination
☐☐☐☐☐ Role player's score
Total mark out of 25

DIFFERENTIAL DIAGNOSIS

Hallux Valgus

Hallux valgus is a valgus deformity of the hallux (1st MTP joint) with lateral deviation of the great toe exceeding 15°. Such angulation results in subluxation of MTP joint of the big toe, which protrudes laterally and becomes prominent, forming a bunion on the first metatarsal head. Friction with shoes may cause the bunion to be swollen and inflamed. It is associated with wide splaying of the forefoot, second digit hammer toe, metatarsalgia, flat feet and secondary osteoarthritis affecting the MTP joint of the big toe. It is commonly bilateral and often the result of inappropriate footwear, such as pointed shoes.

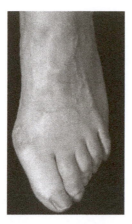

Pes Planus (Flat Foot)

Flat foot is the obliteration of the medial arch of the foot that persists through childhood and into adolescence. Commonly the condition is asymptomatic, but a visible abnormality may be noticed by concerned parents. They may note that their child has an awkward gait and wears shoes poorly. Adults may complain of foot strain or aches in the feet after prolonged walking or standing. On examination, the medial arches of the feet are absent. The patient should be examined whilst sitting to observe for sites of tenderness and range of movement. Particular attention should be spent looking at the individual's shoes, which may reveal excessive wear along the medial border of the sole and outer side of the heel. A complete examination should include the knees, hips and spine to exclude an underlying disorder.

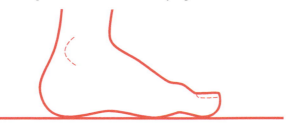

Pes Cavus (High-arched Foot)

Pes cavus describes a higher than normal medial arch. It is often associated with clawing of the toes and varus deformity of the heel. Pes cavus is normally idiopathic; however, neurological disorders such as Charcot–Marie–Tooth disease, Friedreich's ataxia and peroneal muscular atrophy should be excluded. The patient complains of pain in the metatarsal heads and callosities may form over the same sites.

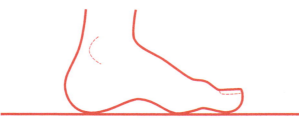

Causes of Pes Cavus

MNEMONIC: 'DISEASE CAN SHORTEN THE FOOT'

Diabetes, **C**harcot–Marie–Tooth, **S**yringomyelia, **T**abes dorsalis, **F**riedreich's ataxia

---

Ruptured Achilles Tendon

The Achilles tendon is a large fibrous cord that connects the calf muscles to the calcaneus. It typically ruptures during strenuous sports activities such as running, football or basketball, which require a forceful push-off with the feet. The patient describes the sudden onset of pain at the back of the ankle, as if they had been struck above the heel. On occasion, a tearing snap can be heard at the time of the incident. On examination, there is tenderness and swelling around the affected tendon. A gap or defect can be seen and palpated 4–5 cm above the calcaneus. There is also associated weakness to plantar flexion of the affected foot, with a positive Simmonds' test.

On the Wards

INSTRUCTIONS

You are a foundation year House Officer in general surgery. Mr Jones is scheduled to have major abdominal surgery in 2 weeks' time. He has asked to speak to a member of the surgical team about pain relief following the operation. Elicit his concerns and explain the pain relief options that can be used.

INTRODUCTION

1 2 3

☐☐☐ **Introduction** Introduce yourself. Confirm the patient's name, age and occupation. Establish rapport with him.

☐☐☐ **Ideas** Confirm the reason for attendance and elicit the patient's understanding and ideas of post-operation pain relief.

'I understand that you are going to have an operation soon and would like to know more about pain relief. Can I ask you what you have already been told?'

☐☐☐ **Concerns** Elicit the patient's concerns, i.e. post-op pain and side effects of painkillers.

'Do you have any particular concerns, about the operation or receiving pain relief? Are there any matters you wish me to clarify?'

Expectations Clarify what the patient would like to know.

'I'm going to explain to you some things about pain relief after your operation. Is that OK? If you have any questions or queries along the way, please stop me and ask.'

EXPLANATION

Pain Relief

Reassure the patient that post-operative pain can be controlled with drugs. Explain that good pain relief reduces recovery time as patients are able to become mobile sooner.

☐☐☐ **Epidural** Explain epidural pain relief to the patient.

'There are a number of ways to control your pain after the operation. This includes an epidural, PCA device and oral medications. I will explain to you each one of these in turn.

'An epidural is a fine tube that is passed between the bones in your back. This fine tube allows small amounts of painkillers to be given directly and continuously to the nerves that relay pain. This tube is taped to your back and connected to a pump which delivers an accurate dose of medication and can be adjusted by the doctor to meet your requirements.'

☐☐☐   **Advantages**   Explain to the patient the advantages of epidural pain relief.

'Because the painkiller acts directly on the nerves that relay pain, smaller amounts of analgesia can be used, so you will receive good pain relief and be less likely to feel drowsy or sick than with other methods. You should also be able to move about in bed more easily and get out of bed sooner than with most other kinds of painkillers. Patients with good pain control progress more quickly and go home earlier. Epidurals are known to be extremely safe and have been used for many years.'

☐☐☐   **Side Effects**   Explain the side effects of epidurals.

'Although epidurals are performed routinely, there is a small chance of suffering from some side effects. The most common of these are relatively minor. You may experience headaches, backaches and problems passing urine. However, you may also experience weakness and numbness of your legs. If you suffer from any of these symptoms and you are worried, please let a doctor or nurse know.

'Although very uncommon, I must inform you that there is a slight possibility that the epidural tube may become infected or bleed around the insertion site. At all times during your stay in hospital you will be regularly checked and monitored so that any potential problems can be treated promptly.'

☐☐☐   **PCA**   Explain to the patient what the PCA is.

'PCA stands for patient-controlled analgesia. This means that you are in direct control of how much pain relief you require for your pain as and when you need it. A special pump that contains the pain relief medication is connected to you by a small tube. This tube may be attached to your i.v. line or your epidural. You control your pain relief mainly by pushing a button that makes the pump deliver you a small, safe dose of analgesia. The total amount of the drug is fixed so that there is no risk of overdosing.'

☐☐☐   **Advantages**   Explain the advantages of PCA pain relief.

'Because the drug enters your body through your veins, it works much faster than tablets. You should feel better within 10 minutes of delivering a dose. This means that you should be able to move about in bed and get out of bed sooner than with tablets alone, and this will help your recovery. PCA is known to be extremely safe and has been used for many years.'

☐☐☐ **Side Effects** Explain the side effects of PCAs.

'Pain-relieving drugs often cause mild sleepiness, nausea and vomiting. Some symptoms are fairly common but can easily be treated. Although the medication should not hurt you as it goes into your vein, you may feel a slight burning or warm feeling. Let a nurse or doctor know if this bothers you.'

☐☐☐ **Alternatives** Explain that there are other forms of pain relief, including tablets and suppositories, once pain becomes milder.

'The epidural/PCA will stop when your pain becomes mild and can be treated in other ways. Eventually, you will be able to take oral medications to control your pain. This will usually be a few days after your operation and may be as tablets, taken orally, or suppositories, through your back passage.'

CLOSING

☐☐☐ **Understanding** Confirm that the patient has understood what you have explained to them.

☐☐☐ **Questions** Respond appropriately to the patient's questions.

☐☐☐ **Leaflet** Offer to give him more information in the form of a handout. Advise that the leaflet contains much of the information you have mentioned.

COMMUNICATION SKILLS

☐☐☐ **Rapport** Attempt to establish rapport with the patient through the use of appropriate eye contact. Maintain appropriate body language and open posture throughout.

☐☐☐ **Listening** Demonstrate interest and concern in what the patient says. Show active listening and listen empathetically.

☐☐☐ **Fluency** Deliver information in a fluent manner. Avoid jargon and repetition.

☐☐☐ **Summary** Provide an appropriate summary to the patient.

EXAMINER'S EVALUATION

1 2 3 4 5

☐☐☐☐☐ Overall assessment of explaining post-op. analgesia

☐☐☐☐☐ Role player's score

Total mark out of 32

INSTRUCTIONS

You are a foundation year doctor in care-of-the-elderly. Mr Dawkins has attended today as his family members have been telling him that he is becoming a little forgetful. Perform an abbreviated mental test score (AMTS) screen and provide an interpretation of your findings.

INTRODUCTION

1 2 3

☐☐☐ **Introduction**   Introduce yourself to the patient as appropriate and establish rapport with him.

☐☐☐ **Name and Occupation**   Elicit the patient's name and former occupation.

HISTORY

☐☐☐ **Problems**   Elicit the patient's awareness of his forgetfulness and memory loss. Elicit the patient's concerns regarding this problem.

☐☐☐ **Explain**   'I am going to ask you a series of questions and ask you to carry out a number of commands to assess your mental state. The commands and questions may appear a little silly but we routinely ask all our patients these.'

ABBREVIATED MENTAL TEST SCORE

One point is scored for each correct answer, with a maximum of 10 points awarded. A score of six or less suggests the possibility of dementia or, in an acute setting, delirium. Further investigations and more formal tests are needed for a reliable diagnosis. More detailed screening tests include the 30-point mini mental state examination (MMSE). Other factors which can lead to low scores include poor cooperation from the patient, English as a second language, hearing difficulties, depression and receptive or expressive dysphasia.

☐☐☐ **Age**   'Could you tell me how old you are?' (Score 1)

☐☐☐ **Time**   'Could you tell me what time it is without looking at a clock?' (Score 1)
The time should be stated to the nearest hour to be awarded a point.

☐☐☐ **Address**   'I am going to tell you an address. Could you repeat it back to me? 42 West Street.'
Ask the patient to repeat the address at the end of the test.
A point can only be given if the patient successfully recalls the address at the end of the test. A point is not awarded for repetition.

☐☐☐ **Year**   'Could you tell me what year it is?' (Score 1)

□□□ **Location** 'Could you tell me the name of the building (hospital/surgery/clinic) we are currently in?' (Score 1)

□□□ **Recognition** 'Could you tell me what my job is?' Next gesture to a nurse and ask, 'Could you tell me what that person's job is?' (Score 1) Only one point can be awarded for correctly recognising two peoples' roles.

□□□ **Date of Birth** 'Could you tell me your date of birth?' (Score 1)

□□□ **WWII Date** 'Could you tell me when the Second World War started?' (Score 1)

□□□ **Monarch** 'What is the name of the current queen or king (or current PM)?' (Score 1)

□□□ **Counting** Ask the patient to count backwards from 20 to 1. (Score 1)

□□□ **Recall** Ask the patient to recall the address stated to the patient earlier. (Score 1)

□□□ **Total** Calculate the patient's AMTS score. (Total out of 10)

□□□ **Closing** Thank the patient for their time and state that you would like take a collateral history and perform a 30-point MMSE if indicated.

COMMUNICATION SKILLS

□□□ **Rapport** Establish and maintain rapport with the patient and demonstrate listening skills.

□□□ **Response** React positively to and acknowledge the patient's emotions.

□□□ **Fluency** Speak fluently and do not use jargon.

□□□ **Summary** Check with the patient and deliver an appropriate summary.

EXAMINER'S EVALUATION

1 2 3 4 5

□□□□□ Overall assessment of performing AMTS

□□□□□ Role player's score

Total mark out of 31

7.3   ON THE WARDS: ACTIVITIES OF DAILY LIVING (ADLs)

INSTRUCTIONS

You are a foundation year House Officer. Mrs Sharone has been in hospital for a month following a stroke that has caused weakness to her right arm and leg. She has been performing well with OT and physiotherapy and may be discharged in the coming weeks. Assess the patient in order to prepare a discharge plan. You will be marked on your ability to perform the assessment and on your communication skills.

INTRODUCTION

1 2 3

☐ ☐ ☐   **Introduction**   Introduce yourself to the patient and confirm their name and age.

☐ ☐ ☐   **Purpose**   Explain the purpose of the consultation.

'I understand that you have been in hospital for 1 month now. The consultant in charge of your care is considering planning for your discharge soon. I am here to ask you a few questions regarding what treatments you received in hospital and what you understand by your condition. I am also going to ask you what issues you think there might be surrounding your discharge home and whether you think any changes may need to be made there. Is it OK for me to proceed?'

HISTORY

*Elicit the Patient's understanding of their situation

☐ ☐ ☐   **Ideas**   Establish the patient's understanding of their planned discharge. What have they already been told?

☐ ☐ ☐   **Concerns**   Does the patient have any particular concerns with her illness or with going home? Find out if the patient has home help or a social network.

☐ ☐ ☐   **Home**   Establish the patient's type of accommodation, and whether she will have to use stairs or a stair lift. Is there anyone else at her home and in what ways do they help her? Was the patient receiving any social services before admission that need to be restarted?

☐ ☐ ☐   **Treatment**   Establish from patient what treatments she has been given.

'You have had a stroke that has left you with a degree of disability. Unfortunately, you will not be at the same level of function as you were prior to the stroke. However, I wish to assess how well you have been functioning in a number of areas whilst you have been in hospital as we can offer some services that may be able to assist you to live as *independently as possible. Is it all right for me to ask you a few questions regarding how you have been coping on the ward?'*

*Assessment of ADLs

☐☐☐ **Washing**   'Have you managed to wash yourself on the ward? Do you require help?'

☐☐☐ **Dressing**   'Have you been able to dress yourself? Do you have any difficulty with grooming such as combing your hair? Do you need assistance?'

☐☐☐ **Mobility**   'Are you able to walk independently? Do you require a frame, stick or wheelchair?'

☐☐☐ **Transferring**   'Are you able to stand from sitting and get out of bed on your own?'

☐☐☐ **Stairs**   'Are you able to manage the stairs?'

☐☐☐ **Cooking**   'Are you able to cook a meal? What can you do by yourself?'

☐☐☐ **Feeding**   'Have you been managing to eat and drink yourself? Do you have any difficulty cutting your food or with chewing and swallowing? Do you require any special food thickeners?'

☐☐☐ **Continence**   'Have you had any accidents with passing stools or urine? Does this happen all the time or only on occasions?'

*Patient's Discharge Needs

☐☐☐ **Carers**   Identify any need for carers to help with washing and dressing.

☐☐☐ **Single Level**   Identify whether the patient is unable to walk up stairs and advise her to seek single-floor accommodation.

☐☐☐ **Shopping**   Identify the need to organise shopping delivery for the patient.

☐☐☐ **Meal Preparation**   Identify if the patient is unable to cook and suggest 'Meals on Wheels'.

☐☐☐ **Continence**   Explain need for a commode next to bed and the use of continence pads.

☐☐☐ **Services Available for Discharge Planning**   When assessing a patient's discharge needs, it is important to know the services each department can offer. The **mnemonic SPOTS** is a useful tool for remembering which services are involved in discharging elderly patients.

Social services	This service can help in a number of areas, from establishing entitlement for financial benefits, arranging carers and services that provide freshly cooked meals, and deal with issues regarding suitable accommodation needs. They can also arrange respite care and can deal with the financial issues pertaining to home modification and care homes.
Physiotherapist	Movement specialists who can help to identify the root mechanical cause of a disability and can improve function through exercise or compensation.
OT	Occupational therapists are able to provide aids and adaptations but also have an important role by working with physiotherapists to improve function, in their case using occupation or functional skills to improve balance, strength and sequencing to ultimately improve rehabilitation.

(Other) **Services**	Other services that can assist include the continence nursing, speech and language (also deal with swallowing issues), district nurses (providing wound care and support at home) and dieticians (assessing patients' nutritional needs).

CLOSING

☐☐☐ **Follow-up**   Offer the patient an outpatient appointment.
☐☐☐ **Understanding** Check that the patient has understood the information provided.
☐☐☐ **Questions**   Encourage patient's questions and respond to them.

THE BARTHEL INDEX

The Barthel Index (BI) or score has been recommended for the functional assessment of elderly patients. It consists of 10 categories that assess a patient's activities of daily living such as mobility, self-grooming and eating. The score is ranked out of 20, with higher scores suggestive of a more 'independent' person. It is a useful tool to assess whether extra services or needs are required for a patient on discharge and whether it is safe for them to go home.

Bowels	Control bowels with no accidents	Bladder control	Urinary control day and night
	0 Incontinent	0	Incontinent (or catheterised)
	1 Occasional accident	1	Occasional accident
	2 Continent	2	Continent (manages catheter alone)
Grooming	Brush teeth, shaving and washing	Bathing	Getting in and out of the bath and washing
	0 Needs help	0	Dependent
	1 Independent	1	Independent
Mobility	Ability to mobilise in house	Transfer	Ability to get up from a bed or chair
	0 Immobile or < 50 metres	0	Unable
	1 Wheelchair independent	1	Major help
	2 Walks with help	2	Minor help
	3 Independent	3	Independent
Eating	Ability to eat food independently	Un/dressing	Ability to put clothes on and take clothes off
	0 Unable to eat unassisted	0	Dependent
	1 Needs help	1	Needs help
	2 Independent	2	Independent
Toilet use	Ability to independently use the toilet	Stairs	Ability to negotiate stairs
	0 Dependent	0	Unable
	1 Needs help	1	Needs help
	2 Independent	2	Independent
Total	Total score out of 20. Scores 0–9: high dependency, 10–19: moderate dependency, 20: independent		

COMMUNICATION SKILLS

☐☐☐ **Rapport** — Establish rapport with the patient and maintain it throughout the interview.

☐☐☐ **Listening** — Demonstrate interest and concern in what the patient says. Show active listening and listen empathically.

☐☐☐ **Summary** — Give a brief summary to the patient about what has been discussed. Jointly agree on an action plan and conclude the interview.

'I am happy to hear that despite your illness you are able to provide help for yourself in a number of areas and you have demonstrated this whilst on the ward. However, there are a few areas in which you need some assistance and I feel we can offer some help. Regarding your problems with washing and dressing, we are able to provide carers who will come to visit you at regular intervals during the day to help you wake up, dress and wash you. As you are no longer able to use the stairs, we recommend you should live on a single level downstairs so that your bed, toilet or commode and kitchen are on the ground floor. As you are finding it difficult to cook for yourself, we can offer a service where we provide ready cooked hot meals for you to eat. We can also organise someone to do your shopping. Regarding issues with continence, we can provide you with pads which should help avoid any messy accidents. We also suggest you place a commode next to your bed in case you need to go in the night. Are you happy with these arrangements?'

EXAMINER'S EVALUATION

1 2 3 4 5

☐☐☐☐☐ Overall assessment of assessing ADL

☐☐☐☐☐ Role player's score

Total mark out of 37

7.4   ON THE WARDS: CHRONIC PAIN MANAGEMENT

INSTRUCTIONS

You are a foundation year House Officer in outpatients. You are asked to see Mrs Kalie, a 45-year-old woman with advanced metastatic breast cancer who is complaining of increasing back pain. You will be marked on the information you provide and your communication skills.

INTRODUCTION

1 2 3

☐☐☐ **Introduction**   Introduce yourself appropriately to the patient and establish rapport with her.

☐☐☐ **Ideas**   Explore the patient's ideas of what she believes may be causing her symptoms.

☐☐☐ **Concerns**   Explore any concerns the patient may have regarding her symptoms.

Expectations   Explore the patient's expectations of what she hopes to achieve during this consultation.

FOCUSED HISTORY

☐☐☐ **Pain**   Ask about where the pain is (site), its severity, time of its onset and character (dull/sharp/colicky or cramp-like). Elicit where the pain radiates and any exacerbating or relieving factors (posture, straining, eating, coughing).

Carcinomas that Metastasise to the Bone

Mnemonic: 'Kinds Of Tumours Leaping Promptly To Bone' **K**idney, **O**vary, **T**estis, **L**ung, **P**rostate, **T**hyroid, **B**reast

---

☐☐☐ **Associated Symp.**   Enquire about fever, nausea and vomiting and pain (in the chest or abdomen). Enquire about fatigue, weight loss, changes in appetite and neurological symptoms (urinary and faecal incontinence, leg numbness and weakness – metastases).

☐☐☐ **Impact on Life**   Enquire how this symptom has impacted on her life.

Experience of Pain

Type	Features
Pleural/peritoneal	Well-localised pain exacerbated by inspiration
Visceral pain	Pain is poorly localised and may refer to other sites (pain is experienced in epigastrium and can radiate to upper lumbar spine)
	Retroperitoneal structures (e.g. pancreas except tail), finds pain worse on lying down and is relieved by sitting forward flexed
Biliary/ureteric/bowel	Episodic colicky/cramp-like pain
Bone/somatic	Often aching, dull and localised over the involved bone. Worse when stressed, e.g. weight bearing. It is typically worse at night.
Neuropathic	Pain can be continuous or intermittent, and experienced in the distribution of a peripheral nerve or nerve root. Pain is often described as stabbing, burning or cold. Numbness, paraesthesia and allodynia are common.

ASSOCIATED HISTORY

☐☐☐ **Medical History** Enquire about any past medical history. Has the patient received any chemotherapy or radiotherapy and if so, how many cycles of treatment? Enquire about the prognosis of cancer and whether there are any metastases. Ask about a history of back pain, sciatica, falls, osteoporosis and disc prolapse. Ask about history of ulcers, asthma, heart and renal failure.

☐☐☐ **Drug History** Establish current medications, including analgesia (NSAIDs – aspirin, opiate – fentanyl patch, morphine sulphate tablets, tramadol, co-codamol, co-dydramol). Enquire about how analgesia is administered (patches, PR, oral, syringe driver). Check patient sensitivities and allergies.

Variable Strengths of Analgesia

Opioid	Dose	Relative (Oramorph)
Codeine	60 mg/qds, PO	0.1
Dihydrocodeine	60 mg/qds, PO	0.1
Pethidine	100 mg/qds, PO	0.175
Tramadol	50 mg/qds, PO	0.2
Pethidine	100 mg/qds, i.m.	0.375
Oramorph/MST	10 mg/4 hrly, PO	1
Oxycodone	5 mg/4 hrly, PO	2
Morphine	5 mg/1–4 hrly, sc, i.v., im	2
Diamorphine	2.5 mg/1–4 hrly, sc	3
Fentanyl	25 mcg/hour	150

☐☐☐ **Mental State** Enquire about how their current symptom has affected their mood. Note that a psychosocial assessment is important, as depression and anxiety are associated with intractable pain.

☐☐☐ **Social History**   Establish her home situation – does she live alone, does she receive help from friends, family or carers? Is she able to get out of the house much? Does she have any contact with a palliative care specialist or a Macmillan nurse?

SYMPTOM MANAGEMENT

Treatment   Discuss with the patient the different options available for the treatment of her symptoms (pharmacological and non-pharmacological) and arrive at an agreed management plan.

☐☐☐ *Non-pharm*   Recommend rest, massages and acupuncture for the pain, and the avoidance of heavy lifting. Consider non-opioid analgesia (TENS, nerve blocks).

☐☐☐ *Pharmacological*   After ascertaining the patient's current analgesic regime, consider optimising pain management by stepping up the WHO analgesic ladder or different routes (intranasal, PR, transdermal, SC).

The Analgesic Ladder for Control of Pain

THE WHO THREE-STEP LADDER FOR CANCER PAIN RELIEF

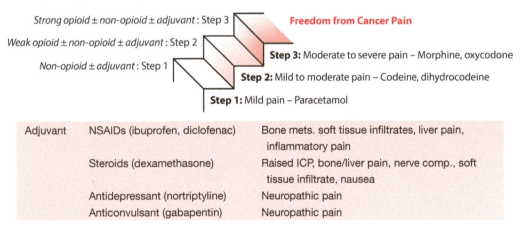

Strong opioid ± non-opioid ± adjuvant : Step 3
Weak opioid ± non-opioid ± adjuvant : Step 2
Non-opioid ± adjuvant : Step 1

Freedom from Cancer Pain

Step 3: Moderate to severe pain – Morphine, oxycodone
Step 2: Mild to moderate pain – Codeine, dihydrocodeine
Step 1: Mild pain – Paracetamol

Adjuvant	NSAIDs (ibuprofen, diclofenac)	Bone mets. soft tissue infiltrates, liver pain, inflammatory pain
	Steroids (dexamethasone)	Raised ICP, bone/liver pain, nerve comp., soft tissue infiltrate, nausea
	Antidepressant (nortriptyline)	Neuropathic pain
	Anticonvulsant (gabapentin)	Neuropathic pain

CLOSING

☐☐☐ **Follow-up**   Offer the patient an outpatient appointment to review her response to treatment.

☐☐☐ **Understanding Questions**   Check that the patient understands the information provided. Encourage patient's questions and respond to them.

COMMUNICATION SKILLS

☐☐☐ **Rapport**   Establish and maintain rapport with the patient throughout the interview.

☐☐☐ **Listening**   Demonstrate an interest and concern in what the patient says. Show active listening and listen empathetically.

☐☐☐ **Verbal Cues**   Use non-verbal and verbal cues, i.e. tone and pace of voice, and nodding head where appropriate.

☐☐☐ **Summarise**   Give a brief summary to the patient about what has been discussed. Jointly agree on an action plan.

'This is Mrs Kalie, a 45-year-old woman suffering from advanced breast cancer that is now being treated palliatively. She had a right-sided mastectomy a number of years ago for her breast cancer. Unfortunately a CT scan of her back revealed significant metastases. Today she has been complaining of continuous pain in her back for the last month that has not been controlled by her slow-release morphine sulphate tablets. She states that the pain is severe and often disturbs her sleep. Her concern is that she will be living out her last remaining days in significant pain. It appears that Mrs Kalie's pain is not adequately controlled by her morphine sulphate tablets. In view of her discomfort I would recommend commencing a morphine syringe driver infusion and have her reviewed in the community by a palliative care nurse to ensure she is comfortable and pain-free.'

EXAMINER'S EVALUATION

1 2 3 4 5

☐☐☐☐☐ Overall assessment of pain management

☐☐☐☐☐ Role player's score

Total mark out of 32

7.5 ON THE WARDS: NAUSEA AND VOMITING MANAGEMENT

INSTRUCTIONS

You are a foundation year House Officer in outpatients. You are asked to see Mr Duke, who is an 83-year-old man with advanced colorectal cancer and is complaining of vomiting and feeling nauseous. Take a history and summarise your findings to the examiner.

INTRODUCTION

1 2 3

☐☐☐ **Introduction** Introduce yourself appropriately to the patient and establish rapport with him.

☐☐☐ **Ideas** Explore the patient's ideas of what he believes may be causing his symptoms.

☐☐☐ **Concerns** Explore any concerns the patient may have regarding his symptoms.

Expectations Explore the patient's expectations of what he hopes to achieve during this consultation.

FOCUSED HISTORY

☐☐☐ **N & V** Ask about when the nausea and vomiting first started (onset), how often it is (frequency) and how much is vomited (volume)? Enquire about the colour of the vomit and its content (bilious, faecal, coffee-ground, blood).

☐☐☐ *Timing* Note when the vomiting occurs. Is it after meals (gastric stasis), or on moving (vestibular disease) or does it wake the patient up (meningeal irritation/raised ICP)? Establish if the nausea dissipates after prolonged periods of vomiting or if it persists. Note that nausea tends to predominate in chemical causes such as hypercalcaemia and renal failure.

☐☐☐ **Associated Symp.** Ask about abdominal pain and distension, time of last bowel motion (constipation – hypercalcaemia) and his ability to pass flatus (bowel obstruction), the passage of urine (obstructive renal failure), indigestion, headaches (ICP), vertigo and tinnitus (vestibular disease). Enquire about weight loss, change in appetite and neurological symptoms (mets).

☐☐☐ **Impact on Life** Enquire about how these symptoms have impacted on his life.

Causes and Features of Vomiting

Causes	Features
Anxiety-related	Nausea occurring in waves or spasms
Motion sickness	Nausea and vomiting on simple movement
Bowel obstruction	Abdominal pain (colicky), distension, worsening nausea and vomiting (vomiting is a late sign in large bowel)
Gastric stasis	Infrequent large volume vomiting followed by relief of symptom. Associated with hiccups, reflux, early epigastric fullness
Gastric outflow obstruction	Associated with projectile vomiting
Oesophageal obstruction	Sensation of food sticking in the oesophagus. Vomiting of unaltered food after ingestion
Chemical-induced	Constant nausea with varying amounts of vomiting
Raised ICP	Early-morning headaches with nausea and vomiting (can wake patient). Photophobia and papilloedema

ASSOCIATED HISTORY

☐☐☐ **Medical History** Enquire about any past medical history. Has the patient received any chemotherapy or radiotherapy and how many cycles have they been given? Enquire about the prognosis of cancer and whether there are any metastases. Ask about motion sickness, endocrine conditions (DM, Addison's), previous reflux, ulcers (*Helicobacter pylori* test), surgery and adhesions.

☐☐☐ **Drug History** Establish current medications including analgesia (NSAIDs – aspirin, opiate – morphine sulphate tablets, tramadol, co-codamol, co-dydramol), iron tablets, digoxin and antibiotics (erythromycin, gentamicin, cephalosporin). Check the patient's sensitivities and allergies.

Mental State Enquire how his current symptom has affected his mood.

☐☐☐ **Social History** Establish home situation – does he live alone, is he receiving help from friends, family or carers? Is he able to get out of the house much? Does he have any contact with a palliative care specialist or Macmillan nurse?

SYMPTOM MANAGEMENT

Treatment Discuss with the patient the different options available for the treatment of his symptoms (pharmacological and non-pharmacological) and arrive at an agreed management plan.

☐☐☐ **Non-pharm.** Recommend small, palatable meals. Suggest he should avoid, if possible, exposure to foods or cooking that may precipitate the nausea. Ask him to consider requesting somebody else to cook for him or purchase prepared foods (to avoid contact with precipitants such as smells). Review his drugs and reduce or stop any identifiable offending medication.

☐☐☐ **Pharmacological** Consider prescribing an antiemetic and describe to the patient the different forms available. Consider oral medication in mild nausea and vomiting (≤ 1/day) and subcutaneous or rectal routes for moderate forms of nausea. Severe or continuous symptoms may require a syringe driver, community nursing or hospice referral.

Choice of Antiemetic

Causes	Antiemetic
Raised intracranial pressure	Cyclizine
Drug-induced/chemical/metabolic	Haloperidol
Unknown or GI obstruction without colic	Metoclopramide
GI obstruction with colic	Hyoscine butylbromide
Gastric irritation	Stop the NSAIDs and PPI
Radiotherapy or chemotherapy	Ondansetron
Multiple causes	Levomepromazine (broad spectrum) – oral or subcutaneous

CLOSING

☐☐☐ **Follow-up**   Offer the patient an outpatient appointment to review treatment response.

☐☐☐ **Understanding Questions**   Check that the patient understands information provided. Encourage the patient to ask questions and respond to them.

COMMUNICATION SKILLS

☐☐☐ **Rapport**   Establish rapport with the patient and maintain it throughout interview.

☐☐☐ **Listening**   Demonstrate interest and concern in what the patient says. Show active listening and listen empathetically.

☐☐☐ **Verbal Cues**   Use non-verbal and verbal cues, i.e. an appropriate tone and pace of voice, nodding head where appropriate.

☐☐☐ **Summarise**   Give a brief summary to the patient of what has been discussed. Jointly agree on an action plan.

'This is Mr Duke, an 83-year-old man suffering from advanced colorectal cancer. He has failed to respond to a course of chemotherapy 3 months ago and is now being treated palliatively. A recent CT scan for his back pain has revealed secondary metastases for which he was commenced on morphine sulphate tablets 10 mg qds and metoclopramide. For the last two weeks he has been suffering from increased nausea and vomiting. The vomiting occurs at any time of the day and bears no relationship to meal times. There is no constipation or haematemesis. His main concern is that he is unable to keep food down and is feeling more fatigued. I suspect that Mr Duke's symptoms are a result of inadequate antiemetic cover for his analgesia and are unlikely to be a result of his failed chemotherapy. I would recommend changing his antiemetic to cyclizine and review the patient's analgesia (start long-acting morphine with low-dose morphine for break-through pain)'.

EXAMINER'S EVALUATION

1 2 3 4 5

☐ ☐ ☐ ☐ ☐   Overall assessment of nausea and vomiting management

☐ ☐ ☐ ☐ ☐   Role player's score

Total mark out of 35

7.6   ON THE WARDS: DYSPNOEA MANAGEMENT

INSTRUCTIONS

You are a foundation year House Officer in outpatients. You are asked to see Mrs Hamlet, a 63-year-old woman with a non-small cell carcinoma. You are here to review this woman as she has been referred from the community health centre because the district nurse is concerned about her increasing shortness of breath. Take a history and summarise your findings to the examiner.

INTRODUCTION

1 2 3

☐☐☐ **Introduction**   Introduce yourself appropriately and establish rapport with the patient.

☐☐☐ **Ideas**   Explore the patient's ideas of what she believes may be causing her symptoms.

☐☐☐ **Concerns**   Explore any concerns the patient may have regarding her symptoms.

Expectations   Explore the patient's expectations of what she hopes to achieve during this consultation.

FOCUSED HISTORY

☐☐☐ **Dyspnoea**   Ask about when the breathlessness started (onset acute or gradual), its nature (intermittent, continuous or exercise-induced), exacerbation and relieving factors (exertion, posture, environmental and stress). Establish whether the dyspnoea affects her sleep (are pillows required, orthopnoea, paroxysmal nocturnal dyspnoea).

☐☐☐ **Associated Symp.**   Do not assume that the patient's breathlessness is directly caused by her cancer. Enquire about wheezing, hoarseness of voice, stridor (airway obstruction), fever, cough, sputum (pneumonia), pleuritic chest pain, calf tenderness, haemoptysis (PE), lethargy (anaemia), chest pain, sweating (angina/MI) or palpitations (arrhythmia). Also enquire about weight loss, change in appetite and neurological symptoms (mets).

☐☐☐ **Impact on Life**   Enquire about how this symptom has impacted on her life.

ASSOCIATED HISTORY

☐☐☐ **Medical History**   Enquire about any past medical history. Has the patient received any chemotherapy or radiotherapy and how many cycles has she been given? Enquire about the prognosis of cancer and whether there are any metastases. Ask about heart failure, asthma, COPD, previous PE and DVTs.

☐☐☐ **Drug History**   Establish her current medications, including analgesia (NSAIDs – aspirin, opiate – morphine sulphate tablets, tramadol, co-codamol, co-dydramol), digoxin and antibiotics (erythromycin, gentamicin, cephalosporin). Check the patient's sensitivities and allergies.

Mental State   Enquire about how her current symptoms have affected her mood.

Social History   Establish her home situation – does she live alone, is she receiving help from friends, family or carers? Is she able to get out of the house much? Does she have any contact with a palliative care specialist or Macmillan nurse?

SYMPTOM MANAGEMENT

Treatment   Discuss with the patient the different options available for the treatment of her symptoms (pharmacological and non-pharmacological) and arrive at an agreed management plan.

☐☐☐ *Non-pharm.*   Recommend breathing and relaxation techniques (positioning, breathing exercises) that can be helpful in controlling her dyspnoea. Encourage the patient to exercise to increase her exercise tolerance. Directing a stream of air (fan) over her face may reduced the sensation of breathlessness. Suggest she keeps the room cool and improves the air ventilation (fan, window). Establish a good position that is comfortable for the patient (sitting upright or forwards eases chest muscles and diaphragm).

☐☐☐ *Pharmacological*   Treatment depends on the suspected cause.

Management of Dyspnoea: Symptomatic Treatment of Dysnopea in Palliative Care

Treatment	Indication
Corticosteroids	Emergency airway obstruction (from tumour or superior vena cava obstruction)
Bronchodilators	Interim measure in partial airway obstruction or as a trial when definitive treatment is not appropriate. Also where reversible airway obstruction is present (asthma/COPD) – consider adrenaline nebulisers for upper-airway tumours
Opioids	Symptomatic relief of dyspnoea towards end of life
Benzodiazepines	Dyspnoea associated with anxiety
Oxygen	Dyspnoeic patients with oxygen saturations of ≤90%

Treatment of Specific Causes

Pneumonia	Antibiotics
Anaemia	Blood transfusions, iron tablets, erythropoietin
Pleural effusion	Pleural tap and pleurodesis (recurrent effusions)
Heart failure	Diuretics/ACE inhibitor
Ascites	Ascitic tap
Airway obstruction	Radiotherapy, stent, corticosteroids
Pulmonary embolism	Anticoagulation therapy (LMWH, warfarin) (remember large central PEs do not present with chest pain)

CLOSING

☐☐☐ **Follow-up**   Offer the patient an outpatient appointment to review treatment response.

☐☐☐ **Understanding**   Check that the patient understands the information provided.
       Questions   Encourage the patient to ask questions and respond to them.

COMMUNICATION SKILLS

☐☐☐ **Rapport**   Establish rapport with the patient and maintain it throughout interview.

☐☐☐ **Listening**   Demonstrate an interest and concern in what the patient says. Show active listening and listen empathetically.

☐☐☐ **Verbal Cues**   Use non-verbal and verbal cues, i.e. an appropriate tone and pace of voice, nodding head where appropriate.

☐☐☐ **Summarise**   Give a brief summary to the patient about what has been discussed. Jointly agree on an action plan.

'This is Mrs Hamlet, a 63-year-old woman suffering from advanced lung cancer which is now being treated palliatively. She has been complaining of a gradual onset of shortness of breath over the last 2 weeks. Over this time she has had a swinging temperature, productive cough with green sputum and some pleuritic chest pain. The patient is concerned that her breathlessness is affecting her day-to-day activities. She has been gasping for air on exertion and is now struggling to climb the flight of stairs to her apartment. I suspect that Mrs Hamlet's symptoms are caused by a chest infection, for which I would like to start a course of antibiotics. However, I would like to carry out a full examination and request for a chest X-ray and a set of blood tests to rule out other potential causes (pleural effusion, pulmonary embolism).'

EXAMINER'S EVALUATION

1 2 3 4 5

☐☐☐☐☐ Overall assessment of dyspnoea treatment

☐☐☐☐☐ Role player's score

Total mark out of 32

7.7   ON THE WARDS: CONSTIPATION MANAGEMENT

INSTRUCTIONS

You are a foundation year House Officer in outpatients. You are asked to see Mr Bowell, who is 65-year-old man with advanced prostate cancer and is complaining of constipation and excessive flatulence. Take a history and summarise your findings to the examiner.

INTRODUCTION

1 2 3

☐☐☐ **Introduction**   Introduce yourself appropriately to the patient and establish rapport with him.

☐☐☐ **Ideas**   Explore the patient's ideas of what he believes may be causing his symptoms.

☐☐☐ **Concerns**   Explore any concerns the patient may have regarding his symptoms.

Expectations   Explore the patient's expectations of what he hopes to achieve during this consultation.

FOCUSED HISTORY

☐☐☐ **Constipation**   Ask the patient what he means by 'constipation'. Ask when it started (onset), how often he passes stools (frequency), its quality (soft, hard) and quantity (large, small)? Enquire whether the stools are painful to pass. Ask if the patient has been immobile over the past few weeks.

CONSTIPATION

There is often a disparity in the understanding of the word 'constipation' between doctors and patients. It is often used by patients to describe painful hard stools or the sensation of incomplete emptying rather than the medical definition of an infrequent passage of stools (< 3/week). It is always important to clarify the patient's own understanding of the word 'constipation' before going down the path of misdiagnosing and mistreating. Treatment is important in order to avoid complications (pain, bowel obstruction, overflow diarrhoea, urinary retention).

Causes of Constipation

Dietary	Dehydration, lack of fluid intake, poor diet (low fibre)
Drugs	Opioids, diuretics, aluminium antacids, iron and calcium supplements, anticholinergics (TCAs), calcium channel blocker
Bowel	Bowel obstruction (abdominal pain, distension, vomiting, tinkling bowel sounds), colon carcinoma (abdominal pain, weight loss, PR blood, mass), diverticular disease, stricture, irritable bowel syndrome
Anal	Anal fissure (perianal tags), haemorrhoids (fresh PR blood on toilet paper, pain)

| Endocrine | Hypothyroidism, hypokalaemia, hypercalcaemia |
| Neuro. | Spinal cord injury, autonomic neuropathy |

☐☐☐ **Bowel Habits** Establish the patient's normal bowel habits, including their frequency, quality and quantity. Identify the presence of altered bowel habits. Ask about episodes of loose stools in between periods of constipation (overflow diarrhoea).

☐☐☐ **Associated Symp.** Ask about abdominal pain and distension, nausea and vomiting, PR bleeding (fresh, melaena) and ability to pass flatus. Enquire about back pain (constant, even at night), weight loss, change in appetite and neurological symptoms (mets).

☐☐☐ **Impact on Life** Enquire about how this symptom has impacted on their life. Note depression in its own right can cause constipation.

ASSOCIATED HISTORY

☐☐☐ **Medical History** Enquire about any past medical history. Has the patient received any chemotherapy or radiotherapy and how many cycles has he been given? Enquire about the prognosis of cancer and whether there are any metastases.

☐☐☐ **Drug History** Establish current medications including analgesia (opiate – morphine sulphate tablets, tramadol, co-codamol, co-dydramol), anticholinergics (TCA – amitriptyline), iron supplements and aluminium salts. Check the patient's sensitivities and allergies.

☐☐☐ **Mental State** Enquire about how his current symptom has affected his mood.

☐☐☐ **Social History** Establish his home situation – does he live alone, is he receiving help from friends, family or carers? Is he able to get out of the house much? Does he have any contact with a palliative care specialist or a Macmillan nurse?

SYMPTOM MANAGEMENT

Treatment Discuss with the patient the different options available for the treatment of his symptoms (pharmacological and non-pharmacological) and arrive at an agreed management plan.

☐☐☐ *Non-pharm.* Advise the patient to drink at least 2 litres of fluid a day and ensure adequate fibre intake. Encourage the patient to mobilise. Also discuss opioid rationalisation – drop down pain ladder or stop offending medication.

Effects and Side Effects of Morphine

MNEMONIC: 'MORPHINE'

Miosis
Out of it (sedation)
Respiratory depression
Pain relief
Hypotension
Infrequency (constipation, urinary retention)
Nausea
Emesis, **E**uphoria

☐☐☐ *Pharmacological*   Consider prescribing a laxative and describe the different forms available (stimulant, softeners, osmotic laxatives).

Choices of Laxative for Constipation

Types	Laxative
Faecal impaction	Arachis oil enema (night), phosphate enema (morning).
Stimulant	(Senna, bisacodyl, co-danthramer) increase intestinal peristalsis but can cause diarrhoea, abdominal cramps and hypokalaemia. Avoid in intestinal obstruction, consider for opioid-induced constipation.
Softeners	(Docusate, co-danthramer) promote defaecation through softening or lubricating the faeces. Safer in resolving intestinal obstruction.
Osmotic	(Movicol, lactulose) increase the amount of water in the bowel by drawing it in or retaining fluid administered with it. Avoid in palliative care (requires 2 l of water to function). Lactulose can cause flatus and bloating (consider pro-kinetic drugs such as metoclopramide and erythromycin).
Constipation	Laxative
Mild	Senna or bisacodyl, docusate, lactulose or movicol
Moderate to severe	Co-danthramer (dual stimulant and softener), glycerine suppositories

EVALUATION

☐☐☐ **Follow-up**   Offer the patient an outpatient appointment to review treatment response.

☐☐☐ **Understanding**   Check that the patient understands the information provided.
Questions   Encourage the patient to ask questions and respond to them.

COMMUNICATION SKILLS

☐☐☐ **Rapport**   Establish rapport with the patient and maintain it throughout the interview.

☐☐☐   **Listening**   Demonstrate an interest and concern in what the patient says. Show active listening and listen empathetically.

☐☐☐   **Verbal Cues**   Use non-verbal and verbal cues, i.e. an appropriate tone and pace of voice, nodding head where appropriate.

☐☐☐   **Summarise**   Give a brief summary to the patient about what has been discussed. Jointly agree on an action plan.

'This is Mr Bowell, a 65-year-old man suffering from advanced prostate cancer which is being treated palliatively. He is complaining for the last 2 weeks of abdominal bloating, pain and less frequent bowel motions. He is not vomiting and is passing flatus. He normally goes daily but recently has been opening his bowels every 2 to 3 days. Recently he has had his analgesia changed from co-dydramol to tramadol. He is concerned that he may suffer a recurrence of his painful haemorrhoids. Taking into consideration his medication, I suspect that Mr Bowell's constipation is secondary to opioids. I would recommend starting a laxative (docusate) and review the patient's analgesia (change to Tramacet). I also recommend that the patient drinks plenty of fluid and mobilises.'

EXAMINER'S EVALUATION

1 2 3 4 5

☐☐☐☐☐   Overall assessment of constipation treatment

☐☐☐☐☐   Role player's score

Total mark out of 36